The Adventures in Vaginoplasty: A Trans Woman's Guide to Healing

By Cristina Michaels M.S. L.Ac.

Table of Contents

Acknowledgements

Although I have never met Dr. Marci Bowers, she was the surgeon that taught the team at Denver Health, where I received my surgery. Dr. Bowers is also a trans woman who is a leader and helped hundreds, if not thousands, of trans people transition. I thank her for all the work she has done to advance the skills of surgeons and dedicate her career to helping trans people. It would be remiss of me to not recognize Denver Health, Dr. Hyers, Shereen, Carli, and all of the amazing support individuals behind the scenes. It is also very important to recognize Morgan Seamont, my loving partner; thank you for your incredible patience and caring assistance during my personal healing and recovery. His unyielding support and help to bring this book to you was beyond incredible.

This gender confirmation surgery is of vital importance to those who seek it out.
I am proud to say this book has had the eyes and hand of trans and queer folx throughout it. I would also like to thank Janet for the coaching and clear insight when my view was clouded and my thoughts scattered. I would like to give a warm hug to all those wonderful women that took part in my surveys. And a special thanks to Jessica for the beautiful flowers and Rachel for her sisterhood.

Be well, Be safe, Stay Flawless!

Introduction

As you use this book, know this is just one way to prepare and help yourself through this incredible journey. Much of this information was gathered over the last seven and eight years from my direct interaction with patients and friends, along with my own personal experiences. Leading up to my surgery date, I spent time researching post-op expectations and recovery. There is so little information out there, it was clear to me that we as a trans community needed something better and more informative. Therefore, while I undertook my own journey with gender confirmation surgery, I took meticulous notes, tried out new treatments and techniques, and put together a book that I think will help others recover more quickly from vaginoplasty.

I have written this book for three reasons. The first is to provide you with a roadmap of what recovery from vaginoplasty looks like. I will cover what you can expect from the first days to the end of the first year, along with some preparation you can do prior to surgery. As a trans woman, I did what most trans women do; I tried to talk with other trans girls who had gone through the surgery. Some had gone through it years beforehand and some had done it more recently, but I always felt like I wanted more information and more details. So, I decided that I would keep a journal of my own experiences, both physical and emotional, to share in this book.

The second reason I wrote this book is because I am a healer. I have over 16,000 hours of experience in massage, acupressure, and acupuncture and have worked closely with various naturopathic healing techniques such as nutrition and healing herbs. In my practice I work with many transgender people and have helped them during their preparation and recovery. I have developed several different techniques through massage, acupressure, and acupuncture to help speed their recovery after various medical procedures associated with trans care, but I will focus primarily on vaginoplasty in this book. I want to share all of my experience with you in order to help you get through the healing process as easily and quickly as possible.

Lastly, I want to share all those little tidbits that your friends and surgeon do not think to mention or forget about. Sometimes that is about recovery, or what to eat, or how to mentally prepare for this exciting and life-saving procedure. These little nuggets might give you the assurance you need that you are not the only person experiencing something, that there is not something wrong with you, or that your surgeon didn't make a mistake. We all had questions when we were recovering from this surgery, and I hope to give you some reassurance throughout your experience. Being assured that others have gone through these things helps to relieve the mental stress of recovering, of having a new body, and of dealing with pains of all sorts. I want you to know that you are not alone. You will learn what to expect and to know the difference between when something is normal and when something is not. You will also learn how your physical therapist, surgeon, and nurses can help you both before surgery and after.

I have added my personal, professional and friend advice and marked it in italicized text throughout the book. I share my own story because I can be more expressive in those sections to tell you my entire experience–both physically and emotionally. In some of those sections you are getting the raw realness of what the experience was like for me or my patients. Please know that everyone's experience is different, and mine might be similar to yours, or it might not. It is important to me that you know as much detail as possible, as this will help relieve much of the mental stress that goes into surgery, healing, and recovery. You need someone to be real with you, and I hope that this book will be one of those sources for you.

Today, transitions can take many different forms depending on each beautiful individual. What may be good for one individual may not be the same for another. This book is geared to the nonbinary and trans-femme individuals who are seeking out, planning for, or have received full or shallow depth vaginoplasty. Within this book, you will find natural and complementary ways to help you heal better and more quickly, while hopefully avoiding some of the common complications.

You should consult your physician to see if they have any concerns about the recommendations provided here. The approach here is to give the reader a weekly OR monthly breakdown of what to expect and how a complementary medical approach to your recovery can provide relief. This is **NOT** a substitute, nor is it a replacement for your physician's advice and guidance. For those individuals seeking overseas procedures, having a physician in your home region who is able to help you if you have any issues arise upon your return can be very important.

The surgery you are undertaking is a major surgery. It is not something that you will go through, spend a week healing, and then go back to your normal life. In fact, you will have to create a whole new normal because everything will be different from now on. Healing will not just take weeks, but months. You will need to be in for a long haul, but it is all worth it! There will probably be days when you question if it was or not, but work through it. We dream of having the perfect set of genitals, but it will take weeks and months to get there. You must be patient with yourself and learn how to care for yourself mentally and physically. It is hard work, but I am here with you to walk through it.

There will be things in this book that may not happen to you; there may be things that do, and there may be things that happen to you that I have not covered. Please note that not all I have written here will happen to you, but I want to be informative about possible complications or side effects, and I feel it is always better to be informed than not know at all. Therefore, take what you need, and utilize whatever materials are provided here. During my own recovery, like most medical practitioners, I started to treat myself as a patient. I researched healing avenues and developed a variety of methods for treatment. I have practiced all of the information presented in this book on myself personally. Professionally, I have also used all of the acupoints on many postoperative patients in my private practice. The results were profound, not just in my patients, but in my own recovery.

The book is organized with a pre-op and post-op checklist. There are some basic recommendations to guide you along your path, questions you should ask yourself, and examples of what things feel like emotionally and physically. In an effort to be thorough, I have broken down the book into different sections covering pre-surgery preparation, the first seven days post-op, the next 14 days, weeks four-six and weeks seven-12,weeks and then it is broken down into three-month segments. There is also insight into 365 days out and beyond.

If you have loved ones around to assist you, there is a Family and Friends chapter to help support those who might be helping you. My hope is to give you a path to healthy healing and a smooth, swift recovery. I have done my best to make this book a simple, user-friendly guide to your new vagina. There is a great deal covered here so let's get started.

Chapter 1

Pre-Op Preparation

I was a baby trans woman at the time when I graduated with my Master of Science in Acupuncture, armed with a spanking new degree and with over 16,000 hours as a professional massage therapy experience. I knew I wanted to find ways to help individuals after their gender-affirming surgeries, be it facial feminization, vaginoplasty, breast augmentation for trans femmes, or chest reconstruction for trans-masculine people.

Initially, many of my patients were trans-masc folks who wanted to reduce their post-op top surgery scars. I quickly developed treatment protocols to help reduce scars within just two visits. I was personally and professionally impressed with the results. At that same time, I had begun researching ways to help trans-femme individuals with their postoperative vaginoplasty pain. Of the few patients I saw in those early days, the results were just as impressive. I knew that Traditional Chinese Medicine could be used in new and different ways to help with gender-confirming surgeries, and to my knowledge, very few individuals were doing this care. I may have been early into my personal transition, but I knew there was a need for postoperative care when it came to my trans family.

During those baby trans years, I too began the mental preparation for my own bottom surgery transition. Years later, and 200-plus hours of relentless electrolysis, my time came. By this point, I knew dozens of individuals who had gone through this procedure, be it in the U.S., Thailand, Canada, or

Mexico. I asked them questions on their recovery. I had also seen some of these folks in my clinic. Using my years in the healing arts, I began to establish what my recovery would look like.

I launched myself into more research, digging through thick Traditional Chinese text books on different healing acupoints. Initially I came up with easy protocols that my partner could administer to me while I recovered. In grad school we were also taught auricular (ear) battlefield acupuncture protocols, and I made sure to purchase the correct needles for that protocol which I could start while I was still in the hospital. I poured over massage techniques, reflexology, and lymph drainage therapies, knowing these types of healing and methods of recovery would in time be passed on to you for your healing and recovery.

Doing Your Research

There are a number of different clinics around the world that perform vaginoplasty. This life-saving gender confirmation surgery (GCS) has options for a full depth or a shallow depth procedure. There are handouts from the clinics you will go to, but often there is little information about what the coming months of recovery will truly look like. Healing looks different for each and every one of us, but there are some norms we will talk about. The full depth procedure will give you a vaginal depth of 5 to 6 inches and a shallow depth procedure will give you a depth of two to three inches. The healing of a shallow depth procedure can be from four to six weeks, while the recovery is four to seven months. The initial healing from the full depth surgery will take six to 12 weeks while recovery will take 10 to 12 months. Healing in the context of this book refers to the physical wounds, and recovery refers to normal bodily function.

Now more than ever, individuals have the ability to pick their surgeons and clinics, as the number of surgeons who specialize in gender confirmation surgery has significantly increased over the last two decades. Some clinics or programs in the United States will keep you for a few days in the hospital, some for 2 weeks and others, mainly overseas, will keep you for 4 weeks. In selecting your clinic and surgeon you will need to consider many factors such as cost, waiting periods, travel, techniques and aesthetics. Those that came before us had to figure out each of these factors, among others, and decide what was best for them. There is no one correct answer. Do what is right for you, but spend some time thinking about these factors and learning as much as you can.

While researching clinics and surgeons, it is good to think about the following:

- Has a friend or community member used this clinic?

- How long will the wait be?

- What technique will the surgeon be using?

- Get clear guidelines on hair removal for the particular technique your surgeon will be using. A visual drawing or diagram is best so you can show it to your electrologist. Also, hair removal can usually be done while you are on the waiting list.

- Ask if you have immediate access to a surgical nurse practitioner or wound specialist when you are sent to recovery. You may want someone you can call to ask about wound concerns or send pictures to in order to ascertain if your wounds are healing normally or if you should come in for evaluation.

- Does the clinic offer physical therapy? Physical therapists who work in these settings can help teach you about dilation (how often, for how long, and when to increase in dilator size), pelvic floor recovery, and also examine the surgical site to ensure everything is healing well.

- How frequently do you get to see the physical therapist during your recovery period? The more often the visits, the better the healing is, in my experience.

- Read information from as many clinics as you can, so you can compare them and ask better questions.

Once you have narrowed down your choices or selected a clinic, here are a few questions you might consider asking:

- Does the clinic or surgeon have a patient who doesn't mind being contacted about how their surgery went? Do not believe everything you read in a blog or reddit post; it is best to go to the source.

- Ask how many procedures they have performed and what their rate of complications is.

- Ask who taught them the procedure and how long their training was.

- How do they handle emergencies during the operation and in the initial stages of healing?

- Ask how quickly they are able to respond to questions.

Beyond looking at clinics, do some pre-op research for physical therapists in your area who specialize in pelvic floor rehabilitation. This might include alternative medical practitioners such as massage therapists, acupuncturists, or pelvic floor specialists. You may need to see a physical therapist more often than your clinic can accommodate. Knowing a few good physical therapists can be very useful if that is the case.

If possible, have a second pair of eyes to read and reread all of the paperwork the clinic will send to you prior to surgery. Another person will also be helpful to ask any questions you may not have thought of or cannot remember because you are nervous and excited to finally talk to a surgeon about your procedure. If you are on a waiting list, get into their pre-op and post-op support groups if possible. These are made up of patients who are either waiting for surgery or have already had it and they can share a great deal of information on what to expect. Get information about the location of the surgery, whether it be a hospital or a clinic. Is there a recovery hotel or housing that is used or recommended by the staff? Sometimes, there is a discount associated with this in a space that offers access to a kitchen so you do not have to go out for food or supplies while initially recovering.

There are some individuals that have VA coverage and will need secondary coverage, since the VA is not currently covering this life-saving surgery. Some states in America have medicaid programs that offer this procedure. There are numerous other types of insurance out there, so please do some research into your own insurance to ascertain what coverage will be like for you.

In my baby trans years, a local hospital where I lived began offering gender-affirming surgeries and there was already a wait-list. I remember that day when I got myself on the list; the excitement was tangible for weeks. Once that exhilaration wore off, I took stock of what needed to be done.

First and foremost, the unpleasantness of hair removal. I did not have the money or the time to do countless hours of laser or electrolysis all at once, nor did I know that it would take 200-plus hours to have complete hair removal. I started with laser only to find out laser does nothing for gray, white, or red hair. But at the time, it was a good place to start. Moving up to electrolysis, I had believed laser treatment was expensive until I found out the cost of electrolysis. I carved out the money and the weekly time of 45 minutes to receive this needle-burning agony. And to think laser treatments were painful!

I remember seeing four different electrologists over the course of three years to finally find the one that worked best for me. I learned that it helps to have a newer machine and to have it cleaned regularly. I learned to ask with confidence how old their electrolysis machine was and when their last cleaning was? I learned there can be over a 50% regrowth rate with cheaper small hand held devices. I wanted it done right the first time, and I wanted the practitioner to be compassionate about the pain that I was putting myself through weekly. Once I got a great deal from an apprentice, two hours for half price. I did that for 30 days twice a week; by the end of the month I was emotionally drained by the 4 hours of weekly pain.

Due to my limited time and funds, the hair removal process went on for two years. Once I got close to having the surgical area cleared of hair, I contacted my clinic monthly for four months before getting onto the six-month countdown list. By this time, I had also learned to sit patiently through the weekly torture. In total, my time on the wait-list was over four years. During that time, I learned about patience, and for me, it further confirmed my commitment to transition in this way.

Hair Removal

Leading up to your procedure, please be especially diligent with your hair removal; do not skimp or use hair removal cream before surgery. Some of the most unfortunate stories I heard were about women who did not fully complete their hair removal and ended up with hair growing inside of their vaginas. I speculate it is very difficult, if not impossible, to remove such hair post-surgically. You have waited a long time for this surgery; please make sure your body is prepared with all of the recommended hair removal done before surgery.

If you have only dark or black hairs to remove, laser hair removal is often sufficient, but not always. At this point in time, electrolysis is your go-to for hair removal. It is time-consuming, painful, and costly. Working with an electrologist who is familiar with gender-confirming surgery and how much hair removal is required is best. If they are not familiar with what to remove, please ensure you get a diagram or a set of directions from your surgeon so your electrologist will be knowledgeable about what to remove. Some gender confirmation clinics will also cauterize the surgical area prior to the surgery to ensure any last minute hair is removed. However, this only works if there are very few follicles to remove. Check with your clinic or hospital.

It is also recommended to not receive electrolysis two weeks prior to your procedure date. This allows the skin to be as healthy as possible. If there are any hairs left at the point of surgery, your surgeon will be able to take care of that during the procedure. So many individuals expect their insurance will pick up this electrolysis tab. Do not assume! Most insurances do NOT cover this critical aspect of transgender care. Do your research.

Also, do not expect to find many electrologists who take insurance. If they take insurance, it may cause a delay in treatment (over a year in some cases). If your insurance does cover electrolysis, you may have to pay up front and then submit a claim for reimbursement. Whatever the case is, do your research, and put electrolysis into your budget to get it done. Once you have completed your electrolysis and selected a clinic, then what?

North America

There are now clinics and hospitals performing this and other gender-affirming surgeries throughout North America (and South America but that will not be discussed here). The wait list for this particular procedure can be long, so it is better to get on it as soon as possible because you can always postpone it if needed. This is also an important thing to ask about when considering which clinic to use—How long is the wait list? Some folks are fine with waiting, especially if there is a particular surgeon they want to use; others do not have that option and must use the one closest to them. There is no shame in that (it is what I had to do) but whatever your case is, it helps to know roughly how long the wait list is. You can use this time to find and educate the folks who will be supporting you in your recovery, put some money aside to live on, and meet the preoperative hair removal requirements.

Overseas

If you have chosen a clinic overseas or outside of North America, you are often there for four weeks, and sometimes the clinic will offer lodging included with the surgery. There are some clinics that will do this surgery for $5000, others for $10,000. Those with the $10k price tag (or more) often come with excellent lodging as well as daily interaction with surgical staff to help care for you. Those who choose a more affordable option may not have the immediate interaction with surgical staff and will have to find their own lodging. Having a safe, quiet, and clean living environment is a **vital** aspect to your early recovery. How clean will the lodging be; will it have daily linen changes? Can you get bedside care and room service? You will need a safe environment and bed rest for a solid two weeks after surgery. You do not need some place that lacks room services, clean linens, and is not quiet. On your flight home, if you can spring for business or first class, your trip will be so much easier. This is a stretch for many of us, but it is well worth the money, as you will not want to sit straight up for the entire flight back. The closer you can get to a horizontal position, the more comfortable you will be.

Ask yourself, will you have someone who will travel with you? What will that look like? What will your return trip look like? For example, if you are flying home from Thailand or Croatia, your return trip could be in excess of 12-16 hours of travel time. There will inevitably be a layover. How long will it be? I've known someone who had to travel five hours home just two weeks post-op. They were in coach, and their trip was agonizing. You will want to plan accordingly for this if you are going out of the country for your surgery. Your travel home will be very important, and you will want to plan out those details as much as possible before your flight so you don't have to worry about them while you are in pain, exhausted, and probably a bit cranky.

Preparing

There are a number of ways you can approach getting ready for this procedure. One bit of advice I was given was to create a Surgery Pre-Flight Checklist. You are the pilot, and you are about to undergo an amazing process, so having a pre-flight checklist can go a long way in making your life easier during this exciting time. Like the pilot of an airplane has a pre-flight checklist to guarantee a safe passage, having your own personal preflight list will help you ensure you are prepared. We will also talk about the in-flight procedures you will need later in this chapter.

Pre-Surgery Checklist

Clear the table of stressful things for the first six weeks post-surgery so that you can heal and recover smoothly. This will be the time you are going to be laying down, resting, and taking care of your new vagina. Define your destination—where do you want to be at the end of your initial healing? You will want as smooth of a recovery process as possible, so what do you need to do in order to rest as much as possible during that time?

Will you have people who can come in and cook meals for you, or do you need to ensure you have enough easy dishes to prepare on your own? Do you have people who can go grocery shopping for you, or will you have it delivered? If you have your groceries delivered; do you have someone who can carry those heavier items? You will be restricted to only lifting less than five to 10 pounds initially, so plan ahead for those heavier items. While you are encouraged to stand and move around during the first six weeks, you will most likely not want to stand for long periods of time.

Easy-to-make meals will be important. Consider freezing meals so you can just pop them in the oven or microwave. Canned soup is another good option; choose ones with low sodium without sugars if possible. Prepared meals are another option, although these tend to be high in sodium, sugars, and preservatives, which will slow down the healing process. Initially, doctors will want you to eat foods high in fiber and/or take a stool softener to ensure you will not be constipated due to pain medication. Doctors do not want you to put any strain on the pelvic floor by bearing down to have a bowel movement, so liquids and fiber will be very important. One thing to keep in mind is that the healthier you eat, such as natural, unprocessed foods, the more you will be helping your body heal from the inside out. Eating fruits and vegetables and naturally made soups will be great.

Prepare for potential boredom during your recovery time. Start a journal to prepare you for the journey. Have your books, knitting, guitar, videos, streaming movies, and shows at the ready. Make some playlists of your favorite music. This is a great time to do those free trials of paid entertainment and then cancel at the end of the trial. Consider downloading some new games or apps to your phone. You could also plan for gaming on a Playstation, Xbox, or other platform, but you will want to remain as horizontal as possible, so ensure that you can lay down. Audio books are another great option during the bedrest phase, so find some good books to download, or check your local library for options. Do you have any hobbies that you can do while laying down? Maybe there is some crafting you would like to do, or other bedside activities.

Focused breathing, meditation, and any form of relaxation such as deep breathing, listening to nature sounds, or visualization will also be great ways of decreasing stress during the healing phase. It is important to set the stage for as little stress as possible. If you are not practiced at these techniques, try downloading an app for guided meditation or breathing exercises to use daily. These techniques will also help you move through the pain you will encounter early on and once you start dilating.

Another way to remove stress is ensuring you have all your finances in order for the six to eight weeks prior to and after surgery. Have you set up ways to pay your bills electronically? Do you have enough savings for food, post-surgery items, and household supplies? Finances are usually a big stressor for everyone, including me, so the more prepared you are to deal with the stresses, the better you will be able to rest and relax.

Lastly, do you have someone to come in and help you, especially during those initial two weeks of healing? You will be tired, in pain, and experiencing emotional highs and lows. Having someone who can help with comfort care, driving you to the clinic or doctor's office, doing laundry, and generally being able to get you what you need will be extremely helpful. Plus, having someone who can keep you company and listen to you complain about your pain, as well as how happy you are with the surgery, is actually beneficial for healing. We are social animals (even if you are introverted), and having some company around–even if they just hang around in another room–is helpful.

If you have a therapist, talk to them beforehand about how to prepare emotionally for the surgery. You will be excited, nervous, and worried all at the same time. Talking about all of those aspects will be helpful. If you do not have a therapist, then talk to a friend, bring it up in a support group, or find someone who has been through this surgery to talk to. Think about what your hopes and fears are and ways that you can address them.

This is a good topic for journaling as well or expressing yourself through painting, drawing, or other media. Writing yourself a motivational letter prior to surgery that you can read when you are down or struggling is another way to prepare. For some of us, a goodbye ritual also might be helpful. Think about how you can honor what you had while simultaneously looking forward to what you will have after this surgery.

Speaking of being stress-free, you will want to have supplies on hand to help you heal. Please see the list below, and add anything else that you can think of.

Things to Get Before Surgery:

- Neck pillow (preferred) or donut cushion

- Outfit to wear home from the hospital, preferably a large dress, loose pajamas, or robe (remember you will have a catheter in place; keep clothes to a minimum)

- Arnicare (gel or ointment)

- Bacitracin (neosporin is not recommended)

- Advil and/or Tylenol

- Pads (long, extra long, overnight)

- Cotton panties that you can throw away when bleeding stops after the first three weeks or so

- Towels or Chux disposable pads to lay on during dilation

- Wet wipes, tissues, or toilet paper for dilation clean up (super helpful)

- Subscription to TV services for boredom relief while taking bed rest

- Books, books, books

- Low-sodium soups for easy food preparation

- Teas to keep you hydrated

- Phone charging cord (don't forget to take it to the hospital and then take it home again)

- Fiber supplement to ensure easy bowel movements

- Hand-held mirror for dilation

- Lap desk, phone holder, and other props to keep your arms from getting tired holding things up

- Slip-on shoes (you will NOT want to bend over to tie shoes)

- Extra pillows for your legs and propping yourself up in bed

Lastly, it is also important to prepare for any potential delay leading up to your procedure. During COVID-19, in the first year or two, there were countless individuals who had their surgeries postponed due to hospital bed shortages. Another gal had her insurance deny her coverage just days before surgery (she was eventually able to resolve the problem). Doctors and nurses get sick sometimes. The point is, delays may happen. Have a plan in place for people you can call or a shoulder you can cry on if it does happen. Use art therapy to process your anger, frustration, and sadness. You will get through it, and you will have the surgery, but if delays happen, you will question that, so have a plan in place if they do.

My wait was nearly five years from when I first signed up for surgery. When I was placed on the six-month list, no one mentioned the possibility of postponement. It had never crossed my mind until that miserable day—three days before my surgery—the surgeon personally called me to notify me that my surgery had been postponed. It was devastating; I still had to see patients that day. My partner had taken time off from work. Things were set into motion that could not easily be reversed.

This was a dark, dark time for me. I had made a pre-surgery checklist, and nothing prepared me for a delay. I tried to find the stainless steel (there was definitely no silver) lining to it all. One colleague had her surgery postponed three times, by the same hospital, during COVID. Her experience brought me hope, knowing I was not alone. I just needed to be resilient, persevere, and things would eventually work out, but initially, I was heartbroken.

I learned quickly from that moment to make some plans (at least tentative ones) for the off-chance that you experience complications and end up spending more time in the hospital than you intended. Do you have people to take care of your pets while you are in the hospital? Can they stay longer if you are still in the hospital? Will the person who is driving you home be able to adjust their schedule? Plan for the worst-case scenario, and then it won't happen.

In-Flight Plan

This is your first six weeks in the healing and recovery phase. Send beautiful thoughts to your new vagina. Imagine the suture and stitches mending without issues and fading away. Foster healing thoughts and kindness to yourself. Set the intention for your healing and recovery. Recognize that healing cannot be rushed, but it can be assisted along the way. Get your rest and manage your pain. Make sure you have your post-surgery instructions from your doctor. Make sure that your caretaker knows what the instructions are as well, as you will tend to forget some of the details due to pain distraction, medication fog, and generally being emotionally overwhelmed. Use all of the tools at your disposal to help you heal and don't be the tough gal who says she doesn't need anything. You are stronger if you ask for the assistance you need.

Post-Flight Plan

As you start back into work life, you may want to question your capacity for the work. Your endurance still may not be back to normal when you have to start work again. You still have 11 to 12 months of healing. Can you take time off if you need a break or work a lighter schedule those first eight weeks back to work? Ask yourself what will you need to touch down in your personal and work life safely? Healing and recovery from this procedure is long and will try your patience at times. Give yourself as much time off as you can possibly afford and know that it will be awhile before you get back to your normal activities. Now that we have laid out what the foundational aspects will be for this journey, let's look at everything in greater detail.

Six Weeks Prior to Surgery

Let's get into your preparation. You will have received a lot of information from your medical provider prior to surgery. Consult that information for pre-op questions, and write down your list of questions for the physician or clinic when you meet them in person. Your body is about to undergo some important and major upgrades and preparing your physical and mental body can go a long way in improving the recovery phase. If possible, six months leading up to the procedures add some stretching, dance or a yoga practice. Practicing Tai Chi and/or Qigong (pronounced Chee-gong) are great ways to prepare your body and mind. Whatever physical activities you like doing, keep doing them! Having a healthy cardiovascular system will also mean less complications and better healing.

Quit all nicotine at least a month prior and a month post surgery–if not indefinitely! This is recommended for all invasive surgical procedures. The use of nicotine can prolong the healing process, prevent wounds from healing quickly, increase your chances of complications, and stymie your recovery. Although there have been no official studies, some patients believe it might also decrease the vaginal depth in those seeking full-depth procedures. If you are addicted to nicotine, talk to your doctor about using patches or medications to help you quit. You can do it!

You may have heard the phrase "We are what we eat." Well, it is time you took it to heart leading up to and after surgery. There are some foods that cause inflammation in some folx but not in others. Inflammation is bad for the body in everyday life, and in a post-surgery situation, it becomes even more detrimental. We will talk more about this in the pre-op inflammation section below, but one important way we can help with inflammation is to stay hydrated. Hydration is important to the body in so many aspects. Keep an eye on your water intake the week prior to your procedure, as it is helpful to your healing. Half your body weight in ounces is a good amount per day. Think of it as adding fresh oil to the engine; your body runs much better when it has enough water.

There are some other ways you can help yourself before going in for the procedure. I mentioned stretches earlier; let's explore that now. Before going into surgery, developing a consistent stretching routine will help your pelvic floor and pelvic region, which will be altered during the surgery. These stretches work a very particular set of muscles that are affected after surgery. While I am suggesting these particular stretches in this pre-op stage, these same stretches will be instrumental in your post operative recovery.

Throughout this book, there will be a reference to these "Pre-Dilation Stretches." These specific stretches are here to help open up and loosen the muscles that have influence on your pelvic floor. They will include some simple pelvic tilts and pelvic floor releases. The first muscle we want to loosen up is the iliopsoas. This muscle can become as thick as your forearm, is attached just below your groin, and runs through your abdominal cavity to your lower back. The optimum stretch of the iliopsoas is done while on one knee. Tuck your pelvis, and gently lunge forward (Image 1).

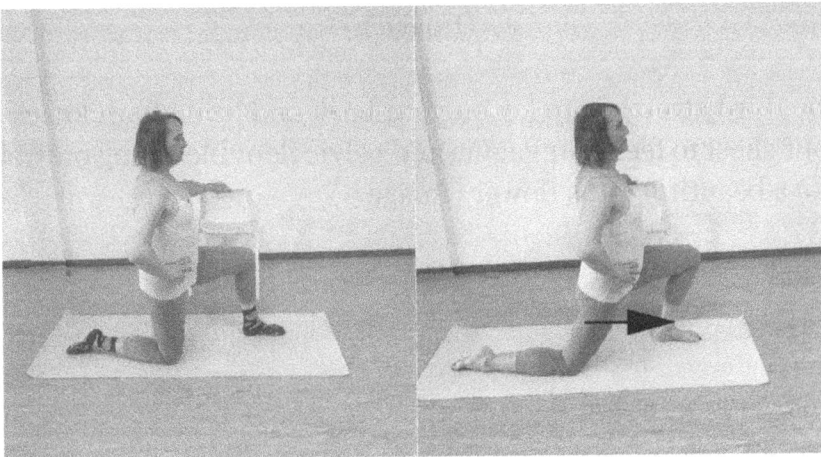

(Image 1)

Hold for two seconds and repeat 10 times or more. The second stretch is an adductor stretch. This muscle group makes up your inner thigh and runs through your pelvis beside the vaginal wall. This stretch is best done laying on your back with your butt up against the wall (Image 2).

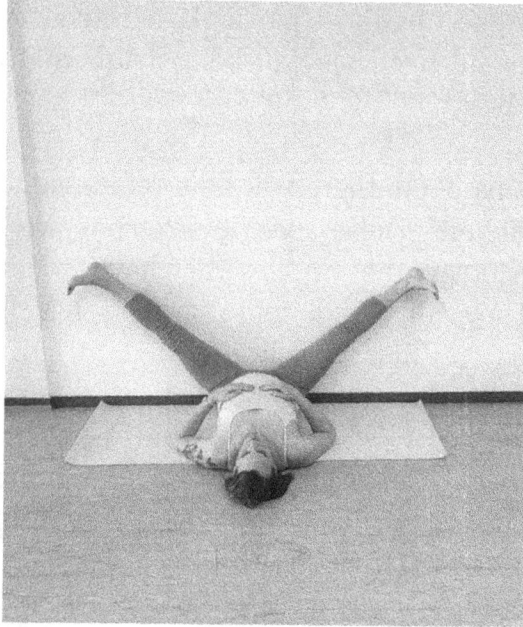

(Image 2)

The third stretch is to lay on your back and bring both knees to your chest to feel your vagina and pelvic floor blooming outward like a beautiful lotus flower (Image 3).

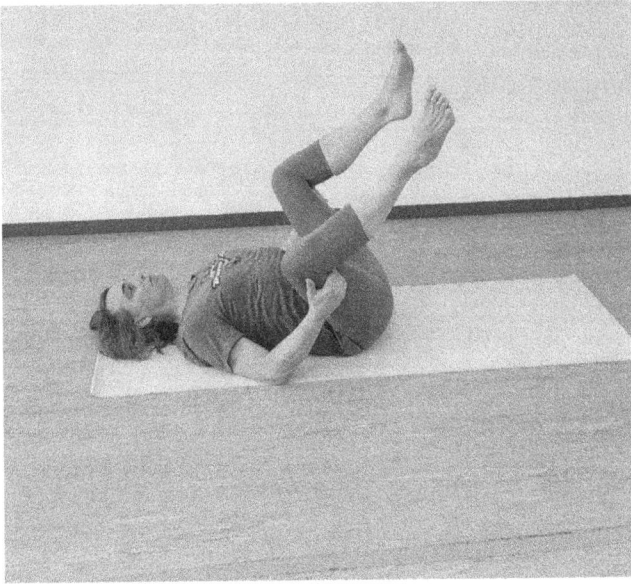

(Image 3)

You will not necessarily feel a stretching sensation while in this position, but you should be able to feel your pelvic floor relax. If you cannot feel this sensation at first, try pushing or bearing down in this position and then relax. This will help loosen the pelvic floor. While on your back, feel free to stretch your hamstrings one leg at a time. You may use a towel around the bottom of your foot, or simply pull your thigh up with your hands behind your leg (Image 4).

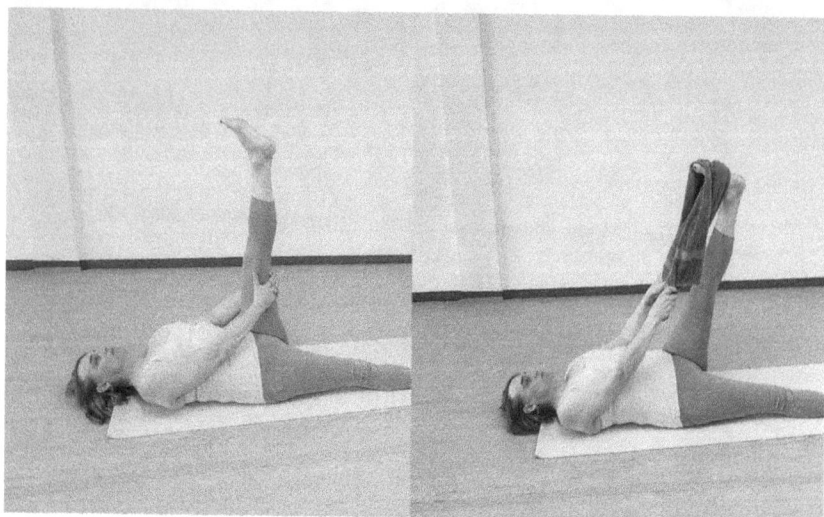

(Image 4)

The last two stretches will also help to loosen up the pelvic floor. Get yourself on the floor on your hands and knees, and take your core and pelvis through a cat and camel stretch. During the cat stretch, you will be flexing your back by pushing your abdomen towards the floor while inhaling and looking up towards the ceiling. During the camel stretch, you will be arching your back by pulling your abdomen away from the floor, exhaling, and tilting your head downwards (Images 5)

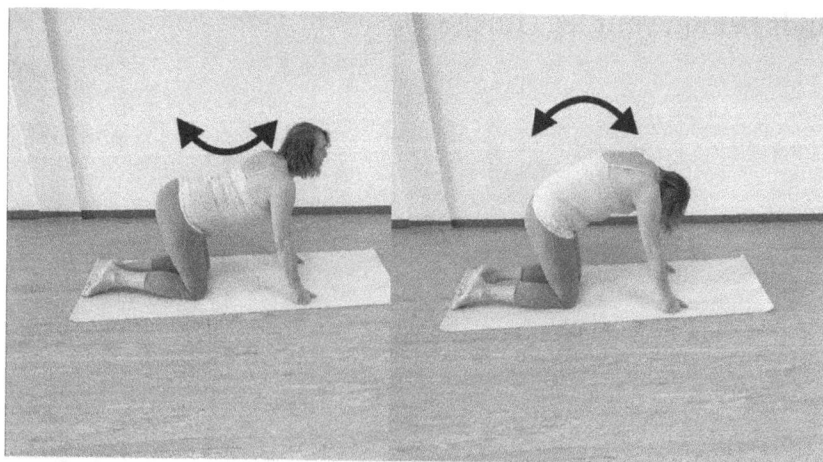

(Image 5)

While standing, practice the pelvic tilt. This action is done by pushing your buttocks out and then tucking your buttocks forward (Image 6).

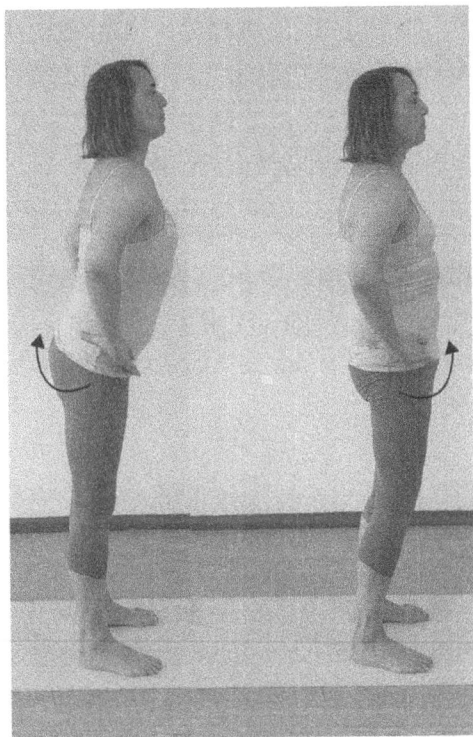

(Image 6)

I have shown the pelvic tilt while standing; however, you can also practice your pelvic tilts while lying down. Getting to know these pre-dilation stretches now can help you in the first few months. From here onward, I will refer to this set of movements as the "pre-dilation stretches." I have listed them below for quick reference. Feel free to dog-ear or bookmark this page for future reference.

Stretches

- Iliopsoas (Image 1) This stretch should be felt in the front of your thigh and groin.

- Adductor stretches (Image 2) This stretch is felt in your inner thighs.

- Pelvic floor stretches (Image 3) This may not be felt all that much.

- Hamstring stretches (Image 4) This will often be felt in the back of the legs. If it radiates below your knee, incorporate some calf stretches before doing the hamstrings.

- Cat & Camel (Image 5) This can be felt in your lower back and along either side of your spine.

- Standing Pelvic Tilt (Image 6) Some individuals may feel this stretch in their lower back and front of the legs.

Pre-Op Inflammation

Why is inflammation bad for the body? When the body has inflammation, there is a particular chain of events set in place. The initial response by the body is to send white blood cells, including granulocytes and macrophages to the wound site or within the body at other sites (the gut is a common one). These give off an array of chemical responses, along with cytokines that are the instant messenger in this chemical response that can kill bacteria or viruses outright. These cytokines then set off another chain of feedback to the body's immune system. Inflammation can come from a variety of areas in your life. So, if the body already has preexisting inflammation such as esophageal reflux, an autoimmune disease or sensitivity/allergies to certain foods, the healing process can become elongated and more complex.

Personal/Professional Note: Prior to my surgery, I consulted a Chinese medical herbalist who was an old classmate of mine, to help me with my internal healing. There are a number of useful Chinese herbal formulas. One known as Yunnan Biayao improves healthy blood circulation leading up to your surgery. This formula has also been shown to support the immune system and promotes muscles and tendon relaxation. The best way to access this herbal formula is through a Chinese medical practitioner or herbalist. I took it for seven days prior to my surgery.

There are foods that have been shown to increase inflammation, so let's take a look at those to ensure we are the healthiest we can be going into surgery and recovery. First, the number-one item is refined sugar. It is in nearly everything we buy to eat, in one form or another. Knowing what is in your foods is a great first step. If sugars are close to the top of the ingredient list, there is a greater percentage of it in the product. Sugar comes in a number of forms with different names: high fructose corn syrup, dextrose, sucrose, fructose, maltose, galactose, glucose, and lactose. They may also try to fool you with brown rice syrup, beet sugar, coconut sugar, date sugar, dextrin maltodextrin, and corn syrup or sugar. Processed foods and fast food chains are some of the biggest culprits when it comes to sugar and preservatives. Such foods have been shown to cause gastrointestinal tract inflammation. There is even sugar in foods that taste salty, so check the nutritional information for everything you eat.

In a variety of individuals, gluten can cause inflammatory issues within the intestinal tract as well. In other folks, dairy might cause inflammation of the intestinal tract. Many of us might enjoy a glass of wine, beer or a hard drink now and then. Alcohol is sugar and should be considered to be within this category.

As a reminder, carbohydrates will convert to glucose in our bodies, which can lead to inflammation. Recognizing what causes inflammation in YOU will go a long way in helping yourself eliminate inflammation prior to surgery, which then allows your body to respond in a healthier way to the changes you are undergoing and the healing your body will need to do. Reducing or eliminating sugar is a great place to start.

Being aware of what we put into our bodies will help in your recovery process. Take a look at your eating habits leading up to your surgery just to give you an idea of how you can improve your recovery and healing process. Foods such as fresh pineapple that have the enzyme bromelain will promote a healthy recovery and are shown to reduce inflammation. The more fruits, vegetables, and healthy proteins you have in your diet, the more healing powers your body will have. All the minerals, vitamins, fiber, and nutrients will provide your body with the materials it needs to heal. See the Help with Healing and Recovery sections below for more discussion on this topic.

Autoimmune Conditions and Healing with Age

Everyone heals slightly differently, but we all have commonalities and similar mechanisms for healing. However, if a body has an autoimmune condition, the body may recover slowly, and there might be more complications with healing. What are autoimmune conditions? Simply put, these conditions or disorders are when the body's immune system attacks itself. There is no rhyme or reason; some may come on early and/or late in age; some may be hereditary; some may seem to have no cause as to why they started. There are some that will be found through blood tests, and others may not be, or your doctor may not test for them. There are a variety of autoimmune disorders. For instance, diabetes is considered an autoimmune condition. These conditions will not prevent you from getting this surgery, but because of the way that they affect the immune system, you may want to do some extra education or preparation. Your surgical staff and anesthesiologist will want to be aware of any potential autoimmune disorders and will talk to you about how that might affect the surgery and healing process.

For individuals with an autoimmune condition such as diabetes, knowing what may cause high blood sugar is important. In the case of a diabetic, when blood sugars go up, it sets into motion a chain reaction of issues in the body. If you fall into this category of autoimmune conditions, being on a low-inflammation diet and being mindful of your sugar intake is very important. This will help in minimizing the inflammation that your body produces after surgery. A number of my family and patients have found that Keto, vegetarian, and or anti-inflammatory eating habits are incredibly helpful in managing their blood glucose levels and internal inflammation. Consult your physician or a registered dietitian six months prior to surgery to get a broader picture of your autoimmune conditions or how you can improve eating habits.

In Chinese Medicine, bone broth and roasted bone marrow is a wonderful way to help prepare the body for this procedure, and Americans are finally realizing these benefits as well. There is a fair amount of blood loss on your surgery day, and bone broth will help build your blood up prior to surgery. Leading up to your procedure, consider making some bone broth soups and freezing them for your return home. I cannot begin to emphasize the importance of bone broth and roasted bone marrow before and after your procedure. In chapter 4, there is nutritional information to help with compromised immunity.

Typically, the older your body is, the longer it will take to heal. Your age can be a factor in your recovery. If the body is not rested, and there are poor dietary habits on top of that, healing will be even longer. A body that is 20 might not have too many issues with recovery. An older body of 50 or 60 may take longer to recover. I am not implying that the younger individual may heal more quickly, either; everyone is different. I am also not implying that if you are older, you should not get the procedure done (I was over 50 when I had it done).

We all transition in our own time, in our own way and that is perfectly fine. With all of this said, I have seen older patients heal faster than younger patients from similar issues. It has also been shown that someone who is active and healthy leading into a procedure will often be quicker to heal. Be mindful of what you put into your body and how much rest you get as we move forward. I cannot stress enough the importance of rest—both for your mind and your body.

Mental Health

Having good access to a mental health practitioner is greatly encouraged. Although I've known a number of individuals who did not have much need for this specialty, they can be useful in helping you prepare for this physical change and what the recovery will involve. I know that we, as a trans community, may have an aversion to seeing mental health professionals due to the gatekeeping nature of medical and mental health. However, this is about going through a major change, both physically and mentally. It is about having someone in your corner to help you get through a very long recovery process. No matter how prepared you are, or how long you have looked forward to this surgery, it is still traumatic to go through a period of healing, of not seeing a perfect vagina when you first wake up, of struggling with the dilation process.

Your mental health is very important to becoming a powerful nonbinary or trans-femme individual. A strong mental frame of mind helps you in your healing and recovery. It goes a very long way to have a professional, licensed therapist to consult pre- and post-op, virtually or in-person. It is also useful to have someone in the role if there are complications, healing takes significantly longer, or other factors you did not plan for come into play.

If you already have a therapist or counselor, it will be much easier and quicker for you to be seen by them. If you do not have access to a licensed therapist, identify pillars of support around you that you could lean on in case you need to. It could be either family, a network of friends, or a partner who can help. A big part of the recovery from this surgery is mental, and having these support pillars will help you considerably. You won't necessarily need it, but it is much better to have some support prepared in case you do.

Sound Advice: One little thing I did was create a living will and a power of attorney. If by chance something went amiss, there were some preset instructions. I was 99% sure nothing bad was going to happen, but having this in place set my mind at ease. And because I am an esoteric individual, I meditated often and sent love and light to all those in that surgery room and the hospital.

Insurance

Insurance can be aggravating to say the least. I have seen them throw roadblocks up for many trans people, and many of them occur right before your surgery date. As some general advice, when you are in contact with your insurance, before asking any questions:

- Get the name of the individual/s you are speaking with.

- Ask for their manager's or supervisor's name and their number.

- Mark the date, length, and time of EVERY conversation or interaction.

- Ask for reference points and locations within their policies to refer to.

- Ask how many physical therapy sessions you can receive after your procedure.

These organizations are providing a service for you; it is your job to make sure they are doing the job for you in the way you need it done. Have any primary questions and secondary questions ready. Ask them where there may be roadblocks (although they may not know). I have had patients get clearance for surgery only to be denied a day before their surgery. This is hard to be prepared for, but know that it is a real possibility. Call the insurance coordinator at your doctor's office for advice and to ask if you should be contacting the company or if they will be contacting the company. Oftentimes, they will speak with the insurance company and ensure that the surgery is covered.

The Friday before my procedure, I waited nervously for one of two phone calls. One would be to confirm the surgery, or the other would be to postpone it again. My ego set me up for disappointment; thankfully it did not happen. Prior to my date, I was advised to wash the night before and the day of my procedure with Hibaclens soap. This may be particular to my surgeon's procedure for pre-op patients. Hibaclens is a way to clean any unnecessary bacteria still on your skin prior to surgery.

After five years of waiting, I followed every detail from the surgical staff regarding my preparation. This included being allowed to have my last cup of black coffee at 4 in the morning. Between 5:30 and 6 a.m., I was allowed about 8 ounces of apple juice. When you had waited as long as I had, I jumped out of the car when we arrived at the hospital; I was so excited to finally be there! Then there is the waiting game; bring a book and your phone to pass the agonizing minutes you are waiting to go back for surgery. Most times, your family or friends are allowed in the pre-op room.

Day-Of Surgery & Hospital Checklist:

What to bring to the hospital:

- Phone and charger

- Laptop and charger

- Powder and Makeup (if wanted)

- Razors (if needed for facial hair)

- Audio books, novels, word games, crosswords, etc.

- Something from home that will make you feel comfortable (a stuffed animal, a special pillow or an extra-comfy blanket)

Turn off your phone and laptop for safety, or hand your phone to a family or friend to communicate your surgery timeline.

Bring a change of clothes, but keep it simple. What you will wear in, you can probably wear out. A simple dress to pull over the head was easiest to manage the catheter on the way home or relocated. Once you are ready to be released, having that easy, over-the-top dress will be a huge help and will make managing the catheter easy.

Some individuals are released from the hospital in three days like myself, while other individuals will be kept for seven or eight days before being transferred to a different living space, so your clothes may be slightly different if you are in that situation. Keeping your clothing to a minimum is best, as you won't want to carry a lot, and you won't need a change of clothes while you are there. Please remember a change of undies or two, and having some clean cotton full brief underwear (light compression underwear) will be easiest and most comfortable. You won't want anything fancy at this point, as you will have blood on your underwear for several days yet. I just bought a whole pack of underwear that I was comfortable throwing away when I stopped bleeding.

Chapter 2

Surgery Day and Your First Seven Days Post-Op

Those last 24 hours leading up to my special time was a mix of overwhelming excitement laced with fear. I needed to protect myself from getting over-excited, so I used the mantra: "I will believe it when it's done." It was similar to waiting for that first time I got to fly. There was all that nervousness about finding the correct gate and preparing, but until I was in the air, I wouldn't believe it. And like that first flight, I was up hours ahead of time. But I had gone through surgery before as a professional ballet dancer, so I generally knew what the process was. I knew that those hours leading up to the zero dark thirty, as I called it, I would be hungry, excited, and tired. Of course that annoying required enema four hours before surgery would wake most people up. I was completely committed and ready to have this done.

I did have the luxury of having my partner there throughout the pre-surgery time. That was invaluable, as the anesthesiologist misgendered me as they asked me about my medical history and preparation. I had waited this long, and being misgendered was one battle I was not up to fighting that early in the morning on an empty stomach. The second time I was misgendered, it was my partner that corrected them on the spot. Oh, the look on that poor woman's face; she did apologize immediately, but having solid support in the pre-op room was a game changer.

The moment I woke up and looked upon my correct body was EUPHORIC! I took the deepest breath possible and just laid there in the glow of it all. My whole groin area was taped up

39

with gauze and bandages. I had a cute little drain tube filled with blood and a catheter tube coming out from under the gauze. It was truly a wonderful sensation.

The surgical staff said that the spinal anesthesia would wear off somewhere between 12 to 24 hours. And at exactly 12 hours post-op, it did! I woke up at 12:30 a.m. with a whole new sensation of pain. It felt like the tip of my former penis had been sewn through relentlessly. I also had a horrible tearing pain in my lower left groin. All of that pain was lessened in about 10 minutes with some meds from the staff and some deep breathing techniques. Despite all the pain, when I would look down there and saw myself in the correct gender, it was GLORIOUS!

The next morning I did what any good acupuncturist would do, and I treated myself using battlefield acupuncture needles known as ASP gold needles. I had my partner insert some into my ear. These dart-like needles are used in battlefield and other triage settings and are meant to fall out within a few days. The use of these particular needles has shown to improve healing by 25% to 30% in battlefield wounds. As a trained acupuncturist I taught my partner to place them in my ears. It did help that he was a former paramedic and familiar with needles.

I had some golden advice from a dear friend when it came to my first walk that came around 48 hours post-op. She said "whatever you do, Crissy, do NOT sit upright on your first walk." I held onto those words closely as it came time to take my first steps. I rolled onto my side to precariously prop myself up. WOW, I did it; I found my feet. But as expected, my center of balance was off a little. I gave out a little chuckle because looking down at my feet there was nothing; there was no bump in the way, just a perfect "v." I could feel my internal *compass pointing to my true center. For me my body finally aligned with my gender.*

There were some steep hurdles to climb those first 7 days. Once the magic trick of 15 feet of packing is removed from your vagina around day 6 or 7, you are shuffled off to the physical therapist to learn how to dilate. My excitement and nervousness took my breath away. When I was presented with my beautiful purple satchel of dilators, I felt like I won an award. That is until I saw the biggest orange one, which looked like it was a rounded 4x4 post. A friend of mine dubbed it "Home Depot."

That first time I inserted the smallest dilator, I had to slow my physical therapist down. It was all so new; I had to take it in, and it hurt a little. For the first time, something was sliding into me in a way I had never experienced before. Little did I know that would be the start of a pretty painful amount of physical therapy in the form of dilation.

Surgery Day

On the day of surgery you will most likely need to arrive at the hospital two three hours prior to your surgical time, if not earlier. For some, it may be very early in the morning; you will probably be nervous, excited, uneasy, and elated all at the same time. You will be hungry, too, as most surgeons will limit your eating before your surgery. My last meal was 12 hours before my surgery, although they did have me wake up at 4 a.m. to drink four ounces of apple juice so my body would have some energy to work off of during surgery. Other surgeons will not want you to have any food the night before. Whatever they suggest, please follow their instructions. If you do eat, they might cancel the surgery because of the risks associated with food remaining in your GI tract and/or the chance of vomiting during anesthesia.

My surgeon also had me do an enema before I left the house that morning. This is important because you want your bowels and anus to be as clean as possible while they are working in that area. Should any leakage occur during surgery, it would greatly increase the chance of infection. Further, there is always the smallest chance that a fistula (an abnormal connection between two structures) may occur between your rectum and the vagina. So if you are asked to take this step, please do so. The doctors are only interested in making this surgery as safe as possible and eliminating any possible chances of complications.

After you arrive at the hospital, you will check in with the surgery receptionist, answer some questions and probably sign some more paperwork. Then the waiting period begins. It is hard to sit still—or at least it was for me. I tried to distract myself with a magazine or watching TV, but finally I just took some deep breaths and tried to focus on giving my body the love it deserved and would need in the next few weeks. *I did pee standing up one last time.*

Finally, the nurses will call you back to the pre-surgery area and your partner, caretaker, or family member will usually be allowed to go with you. You will be asked to change into a gown and get into a hospital bed. Nurses will ask you lots of questions related to your medical history, medications and prepare you for surgery by starting an IV and giving you any medications you will need. Once they are done, your anesthesiologist will come in and ask you some more questions—and probably some of the same ones you were already asked. Your surgeon will also come in and check in with you, answer any last minute questions you might have. This all seems to take forever, especially when you just want to get everything going! Have patience, take some deep breaths, and ask for another warm blanket (this was one of the best parts of the pre-op area!).

I feel like this next part is an important aspect of surgery that doesn't get talked about very often, so let me pause and take a minute to delve more deeply into it. I have mentioned that I am an esoteric soul. And this is not something many trans folx may want to discuss. But as I waited patiently, I thanked my body for all that it had done up to this point. I told my body I was about to ask a big favor from it. I may not have wanted my penis, but a final thank you and a kind, loving goodbye was in order. It was the very least I could do. It had stood up accordingly, no pun intended. I may not have wanted my penis, but it was part of me and so I wanted to acknowledge the loss even while I was wanting it gone.

When it gets really close to your time, the hospital area may sound and look like a well-organized rush hour. Everyone is busy, busy, busy. You are given your last dose of medicine and wheeled away to the operating room. I had never been given a spinal tap, so be ready for that if it will also be a new experience for you. The attending anesthesiologist or assistant will numb the area prior to your spinal tap.

I remember looking and focusing intently on my surgical staff assistant's eyes and gripping their hands as that spinal entered my body. You will feel your legs go numb, and you will get really sleepy. Now comes the easiest part of your hospital stay, as you are asleep the entire time. This will also be one of the most stressful times for your partner, caretaker, or family member. My surgery took about four hours and another three in recovery, which is a long time for your loved ones to sit and wait to hear how things went and if everything is OK. Luckily, it was my surgeon's policy to give regular updates to my partner while I was in surgery. So, periodically, he was called and told that I was doing fine and that the procedure was going well. It was a relief to him and helped his own nervousness too.

When I woke at first, I almost didn't believe it was over. It appeared that I was in the same room I was in before surgery. I was groggy as I looked around the space. I immediately looked down at my groin and slowly pulled back the covers. The sigh that I released that moment could have been heard throughout the hospital. I was elated and exhausted at the same moment. The harmonious hum that settled upon my psyche was one of rebirth and love.

After you are done in recovery, they will move you to a regular hospital room. You will be feeling much more awake by this point and will move into a more comfortable hospital bed. Your IV will remain in place while you are in the hospital in order to give you fluids, antibiotics, and other medication as needed. Your caregiver will be able to come and see you at this point, which is always a relief to the both of you. As I said earlier, this is a big surgery, and while the possibility of complications happening is very low, you will both still worry, and it is nice to have them by your side. At this point, if you were given a spinal block, your pain will be minimal, if at all. You may look a little pale at first, but some rest and some light food will help that. While you can't directly see your groin because of all the tape and bandages, you will still be very excited to see the change!

Many of you will experience a lot of emotions those first few hours and days post-op. Euphoria, grief, excitement, relief (and many more emotions) may come into play. Let the emotional wave be part of this ride. No matter how well you prepare, recovery can be an emotional roller coaster. This is the time for you to rest, heal, and recover. If you're tired, sleep. And you will get tired easily in these first few days. It is best to listen to your body and sleep if it wants to. Sleep is when a lot of healing takes place, so take advantage and get as many naps as you can. Limit the amount of visiting you do with people; you will run out of energy quickly.

A drain tube will be in place to help remove any excess blood and fluid from your surgical site. A catheter will be in place to empty your bladder of urine, and keep the surgical site clean and uncontaminated. The drain will be removed within 2-4 days and the catheter will be removed in about a week. On your legs will be a circulation helper. These helpers squeeze your legs by inflating with air, periodically those first few days. They help prevent blood clots from forming as you are on strict bed rest for the initial 72 hours.

There will be a moment when the spinal tap wears off, and it will be different for everyone. I spoke to a few individuals after the fact who said they did not experience any pain when the spinal wore off. *In my case, that could not be farther from the truth. I woke up at 12:30 a.m. in the most excruciating pain. I could feel nearly every suture and incision in my body. I could not differentiate from the tearing pain or the overwhelming sensation like someone had sewn repeatedly through the top of my former penis. There was a tearing sensation to the left of my surgical site that left a psycho-emotional mark on me for a few months. It took lots of self-massage and acupuncture to alleviate that deep, unseen wound. I will go further into caring for those and other issues that may arise in later chapters.*

Helping Yourself Through Recovery

Bromelain is an enzyme that comes from the pineapple plant; it is also known as pineapple extract. Pineapple extract is mother nature's natural anti-inflammatory; it comes in pill or capsule form. You can find it at your local natural grocery store. Bromelain is wonderful at decreasing bruising and reducing inflammation, but like any wound, it takes time and care to heal from surgery. I suggest taking it the second day out of surgery. I also took it five days before my surgical date. I brought it into the hospital with my usual supplies (cell phone charger, laptop, and book). You may take it on an empty stomach; it is not hard on our digestive tract. If you are allergic to pineapple, I would not suggest it, of course. If eating pineapple directly–rather than taking the extract–use only fresh pineapple, not canned or processed. I also would not rule out the benefits of turmeric tablets as a way to reduce inflammation. In my professional practice, I have seen wonderful results in combination with bromelain.

Bromelain Tidbit: I once had an individual tell me that they were at a wedding and accidentally had eaten something with shellfish. Their throat began to close up, and they started having breathing issues. It just so happened that in the buffet line were fresh cut pineapples. Without thinking, they just started eating the fresh pineapple. Within less than a minute, their throat cleared, and their breathing issues had decreased. They did eventually get an Epipen to assist them with the allergic reaction. They had no idea that pineapple was an anti-inflammatory.

The next few days in the hospital follow a routine of rest, managing pain, trying to eat something, drinking plenty of water, exercising your lungs with a spirometer, and boredom. You will be given a spirometer that is used to strengthen your lungs and cardiovascular systems. I would highly encourage you to bring the spirometer home with you to continue to strengthen your lungs and help prevent coughing and pneumonia. Most hospitals will want you to use it every hour.

Listening to what the medical practitioners say at this point is important. This is when you need to rest. You will be happy to have brought a book, have some music to listen to, games to play on your phone, audiobooks, or a TV to watch. Again, short visits from people is fine, but go easy, and feel free to tell them that you need to get some rest. Hospital staff will not want you to get out of bed initially. If you need to get out of bed after they have given you the OK to do so, make sure to call for a nurse beforehand so they can help manage your catheter, your IV, and help steady you so you do not fall. However, they will most likely have you use a bedpan rather than get out of bed as you should not be on your feet.

It is important to start to manage your pain during your hospital stay. It is called "staying ahead of your pain." What does this mean? If you wait too long to take medication for your pain, then it won't work as well because your pain level is too high. If you take it as directed–usually every four hours to begin with–you end up taking the medication before your pain gets really bad. This will allow you to stay on top of your pain rather than waiting until it gets really bad and being behind your pain. This will be important when you go home too, so practicing now will help you over the next few weeks.

Around day three, you will be asked to take a short walk. Short is the operative word here. Make sure you go slow. Moving will actually help things heal and get more blood flow to the area, which will help decrease swelling and prevent blood clots. One thing to remember is that your pelvic floor has just been completely remodeled and upgraded! You will need to learn to do things differently now. <u>Please do your best to **not** sit up in bed</u>. I would suggest rolling onto one of your butt cheeks and propping yourself up until you can get your legs and feet onto the floor. Sitting upright will be extremely painful, and you probably don't want that.

The day I was released from the hospital was when my bandages came off, and the drain was removed (but not the catheter). Now is the time to put on a fresh pair of cotton underwear. You will want to have a thick overnight pad for your drive home. That first time you pull up your underwear is

47

simply breathtaking. I still remember that incredibly profound feeling that afternoon; there was definitely a foreign feeling as I slid the undies on. But that new feeling gave me strength and deep reassurance in those first few moments. I finally had the body I was meant to have.

The Trip Home

You will want to think about the trip home ahead of time. It is best if you can lay down during the car ride home, so take a look at the car you will be using. Can you lay down in the back seat? Can the front seat recline all the way? You will want a pillow to sit on, whether it is a neck pillow, a donut pillow, or a regular pillow. You will probably want to take some pain medicine about 30 minutes before you leave in order to make the trip more comfortable, especially if you have a long way to travel.

This is also where an easy, loose-fitting dress comes in handy. Having something that you can just slip over your head is easiest and will allow you to manage the catheter tubing without feeding it through your pant legs. It will help at home to have something you can just slip out of when you climb into bed, or simply wear a dress that you can sleep in.

Once you get going, there really isn't anything to do but grit your teeth, breathe, and bear it as best you can. No matter how smooth your driver tries to be, the road is a lot bumpier than you ever thought it was. Try to tilt slightly onto one of your butt cheeks if the pressure on your vaginal area is too intense. You can also use the hand hold located above the door in many cars to lift some of your bodyweight off of your pelvis to ease the pressure. Breathe through the discomfort, and think of how nice it will be to get home.

Once you are home, you will probably just want to crawl into bed. Make sure you have everything you need around you if your person is leaving. Just like in the hospital, you will want some water, tissues, your phone, your tablet or computer, and it is helpful to have a bucket nearby for your catheter. Having a few Chux pads to put on the bed to catch any bleeding that may happen during the night will be useful as well. You will have been given directions at the hospital on when to empty your catheter or how to measure the amount of urine output (if needed). If you don't have the energy to get up, your caretaker can simply empty the contents into the bucket and then carry it to the toilet.

Hydration

One good aspect of having a catheter in is, you do not have to worry about going to the bathroom as often, so slowly start some post-op hydration. Some juice, water, or broth will help the digestive actions of the intestines to reactivate. Have some juice while in recovery those first six or seven days, but do not make it your only fluid, as it is high in sugar. Consider some bone broth soup (see the section below). Inflammation can get worse, and healing can take longer when you are dehydrated.

I like to recommend to my patients to drink around half their bodies' weight in ounces daily. An example is, if an individual weighs 170 pounds, they would drink roughly 85 ounces a day. This would include herbal teas, unsweetened juices and water. You will not need to drink this much while you are in the hospital, as you will be receiving some IV fluids. As you go home and begin recovery in your own space, it is important to ensure you get enough fluids. If your urine is very dark, you are not drinking enough. Teas are also an excellent way to ingest more liquids, especially herbal tea without caffeine. Keep hydrating more than usual for the first six weeks, as it will help keep your circulatory system to remove swelling from the surgery area.

Now that you are home, you will still want to stay as horizontal as possible for the next few days. REST, REST, REST. This is your job—Do it well. This is when you will need the most help at home. Have someone bring you food. Soup is a great starting point as it will help you hydrate, is very nutritional, and makes for easy bowel movements.

Speaking of bowel movements, you will probably be wanting to have one (or might have had one already before leaving the hospital). Know that some pain medications they may give you in the hospital may cause constipation. You will be sent home with some stool-softening medication; please take it as prescribed unless you are suffering from diarrhea. *For me, when I took the stool softener, it actually made me have horrible, continuous diarrhea, which is not something you want, either.* You do not want to bear down, push down, or strain during a bowel movement, especially while the packing is still in place.

These first seven days, it may help to look at the surgical site as a wound site. You will not be seeing the perfect set of genitals when you first get the opportunity to look at the surgical area. It might even be scary to look at all of the open wounds. The medical staff recommended an antibacterial ointment for the surgical site. It will help to apply it throughout the day this first week. It will also help to have at least three or four tubes of bacitracin at home that first week.

Even though you will be resting a lot, it is important to get up several times a day and move around. Take short walks throughout the day to keep the blood moving, which will help with the swelling and moving lymphatic fluid out of the area. Plus, it will help to break up the boredom. These walks do not need to be long or fast; short and slow is just fine. They will also help to prevent any potential blood clots developing from laying in bed and resting. In the next few days, you will be able to empty the catheter bag yourself. This might be done more easily while standing up rather than sitting down. This was strange, as I had been sitting down to pee for years, and suddenly, after I had gotten my vagina, I was going backward and standing up to pee! It was funny to me. But seriously, it is easier to hold the foley bag over the toilet while standing and empty it that way.

The first four days home, it was an enormous help to have someone empty the foley bag, make me food, and generally fetch things as needed for me; it made a big difference. Sitting is nearly out of the question, unless you have lots of pillows and you're at a slight angle. Lying on your side will be a common position these first few weeks. Let pain be your guide. Rest, recover, and send beautiful, healing thoughts to your new vagina. Those first few days can be tough.

Showers

After not having a shower for a few days in the hospital, it will be nice to take one and get cleaned up. Those first seven days showering may seem intimidating. Do not scrub over your wounds! Use soap to lather up above, and let the water to naturally go where gravity takes it. You can clean your bum just fine, but you will feel the inflammation in the perineal space. Be gentle. You will use the shower as your normal cleaning cycle for the non-surgical areas of your body. You will be using a sitz bath for keeping your vagina clean after you get the OK from your surgeon.

On day six or seven, you will return to the surgeon's office to finally get the packing taken out, the Foley catheter removed, and have the surgical site checked. I will tell you now that the removal of the packing was an unpleasant experience for me, and I felt like a clown with someone removing yards and yards of the stuff out of my new vagina. On the other hand, it felt so good to have it gone. After they take the packing out, they will prepare you to test your bladder.

It is time to make sure your ureter is functioning. This means that they disconnect the bag from your catheter line. Prior to the full removal of your catheter tube, the doctor will fill your bladder with a sterile saline solution. They will then remove the catheter tube and have you go pee. For me, I don't ever remember scrambling so fast to go pee (while moving so slow); you may feel like you will explode. They will measure the amount of urine you release to make sure the fluid they put in is the same amount you let out. Due to inflammation at your surgical site and the shortening of your urethra, you will find that your urine stream will change over the course of the next 12 weeks. There are so many stories about trans women spraying or peeing on their legs or outside of the toilet bowl. *They are all true!* You can try tilting your pelvis up and down to see if that changes the stream(s), but be prepared for an unusual experience—You will never know until it comes out.

The surgeon will examine your wound site and make sure everything is looking OK. They will answer any questions you might have as well, so be sure to write them down and bring them with you to this appointment. As long as everything is healing as it should, you will then be sent to the physical therapist who will assist you in learning how to dilate.

This is an awkward and exciting moment all at the same time. At this point, I was fairly used to opening up my legs and letting yet another person look at me and poke and prod around. However, my physical therapist was very respectful of what I wanted and how I was feeling—It was a nice change of pace. She first showed me the dilators, talked about which one to use, how to clean them, etc. And then came the moment of truth, when something was going to enter my vagina for the first time. She asked if I wanted to insert the dilator or if I wanted her to do it. I asked her to do it because I was pretty nervous about it—I didn't want to break my new vagina by pushing too hard or something.

She showed me how to lube it up and had me watch what she was doing with a mirror so I could learn how to do it. Due to the particular skin used for the vagina the sensation of inserting the dilator was fascinatingly confusing. It will take some time to get used to the beautiful new sensation. Your body has had a steep learning curve over the last few days. Not only has your immune system been diligently healing your physical body, but your brain is adjusting to all sorts of new sensations. Be patient and listen to your body during all of your phases of healing.

Now that you are done with your first post-op visit it is time to go home (a much easier process now that your catheter and packing are out), and start really managing your wound care, which is what we will be talking about in the next chapter.

Sound Advice: As a dear friend once told me, "That first month, all you are doing is caring for your new vagina." I took it to heart, as should you.

This procedure is lifesaving for those who can receive it, but the first few months can be hard at times. In an effort to look at myself and my patients' vaginoplasty as a facet of healing, I chose those first six weeks to look at this procedure not just as a neo-vagina, but also as a wound and surgical site.

I do not speak for all trans women, but for many of us, we typically spend years (if not decades) envisioning what our bodies will look like after surgery. In our heads, we are probably picturing the perfect vagina, the perfect clitoris, the perfect labia–whatever that is for each of us. What we are unaware of is how our genitals will look while we are healing, and especially during the first few days/weeks when nothing has healed yet.

For the first few weeks, it will look like a bad wound–a really bad wound. Let's be totally honest about what your vagina and vulva are going to look like after surgery. At first glance, you will have excitement to finally see the correct profile. It will also look and feel like someone took a chainsaw to your groin. It may be slightly unnerving to see it. You may wonder if you made a mistake. Take a deep breath, and know that things will heal beautifully. It will get better, and it will get prettier, but it will take some time. Be patient with yourself, and do what you can to make sure your body is getting what it needs in order to heal as fast as possible and to avoid any complications.

*Sound Advice: Although this is broken down into the first seven days and then the next 14 days, those first two weeks are when you will **need the most assistance**, so plan accordingly. Weeks three through four will become <u>slightly</u> easier to get around the living space. For me, my partner had to go back to work after two weeks, and that is the week I had asked friends and family to bring me prepared foods. Please refer to the Friends and Family section.*

Chapter 3

Week Two and Three

The specific clinic that I used was Denver Health; they had a transgender care team that was in regular communication with one another. For instance, if I reported a problem to my physical therapist about wound care, my surgeon and her nurse practitioner were also informed. This reassured me that the whole team knew what I was going through. They stepped in and requested that I see them when it was necessary. The team was also there for me as I moved from surgery to recovery to hospital release. For example, my surgeon checked on me in the immediate hours after surgery in POCU, (Post-Operative Care Unit). POCU is one step down from Intensive Care.

In the hours and days that followed, the head nurse practitioner was the key point person. By the end of the first week, I saw the head nurse practitioner and the physical therapist. Every 10 days, I saw the physical therapist, and at three weeks, I saw the surgeon again and the nurse practitioner. If something arose, I had access to the surgeon, often within hours. The physical therapist had their eyes on any infection and surgical site concerns with me every 10 days or so.

This ongoing teamwork lasted up to four months in my case. The team was also very communicative with my caregiver and partner as well. Forty-five minutes into surgery, a team member called my partner to inform him where they were in surgery and how I was doing. At 120 minutes, he got another call on my progress; at around three and a half hours, he got another call. When going overseas or within North America, inquire if you will have a team, and who is your team? Will you have immediate messaging with a nurse practitioner or a wound specialist, or will you need to call the provider and wait for a return call?

Sometimes, in spite of all the preparation we have done, there are complications. Around day nine, something very serious and worrying happened to me. It had become painful to dilate, and there was some dark yellow or gray skin hanging from my vagina. Now, the first thing I thought was that my graft had failed. I was mortified. But then, how was I able to still dilate, and there was no fever and no infection symptoms? This hanging skin was freaking me out! The surgical staff told me when I was released that if I had some concerns, I could snap a photo of my vajayjay and send it to them via the health system email. The last thing I wanted to do was take a photo of my vajayjay, but I did!

The same day, I was seen by the surgeon to have her snip away this skin. Now, I did not have a view of said "snipping," but I watched my partner's eyes get big as saucers as the surgeon did it. He added hesitantly, "So, you don't need a local anesthetic for that?"

"Nope." said the surgeon sincerely, adding, "It is all just dead skin; in her case it just came off sooner."

I will say, I have had patients call me in a panic about this same issue. This is why I have placed this warning at the beginning of this chapter. I was lucky that the tissue was not infected, and I had no infection in other parts of the surgical area, but infection is important to talk about in more detail. Learning to recognize an infection is important. There is a lot going on in your first 21 days; read it twice to prepare yourself. Or just read it while you heal in bed.

Wound and Surgical Site Infection

Let us start with the most obvious question. What is the best way to keep a wound clean? If you cut your finger deeply, you would wash it, wrap it up, keep it clean and disinfected. Your **NUMBER ONE** priority these first eight weeks is to keep your newly renovated genitalia clean, cared for, and protected from infection. This is very important. You do not want to experience infection or other problems that could affect your new vagina.

What does an infection look like? Redness, soreness, and/or abnormal swelling in the area of surgery along with a fever. Pain or burning sensation when urinating is a sign of a urinary tract infection. Unusual vaginal discharge or excessive bleeding can also be a sign that your wounds are infected. This can be difficult to notice in the early stages of healing, so pay close attention to any fevers. If you are concerned, you should call the nurse at your surgeon's office for an examination. If you notice red streaking on your skin moving out from your surgical site or have a high fever, you should call your surgeon immediately or go to the emergency room.

Swelling and Bruising

After surgery, there will be a tremendous amount of swelling and bruising of the inner thigh, lower abdomen, and anywhere around the pelvic area and rectum. Have your ice pack ready. We will be talking about swelling throughout the book, but I will address it more specifically here.

Arnica

Arnica ointment and gels are derivatives from the Arnica plant, which can help with localized bruising, swelling, and general inflammation. This ointment, or gel, is for EXTERNAL use only. Only apply it to the healthy skin surrounding your new vagina. Do not apply it directly to any wounds. There are a number of companies that sell some form of Arnica ointment or gel. Applied to the skin, this product helps marvelously with bruising, swelling, and inflammation. You do not need a lot and oftentimes it can be added to small amounts of massage oil to help massage it in.

From my personal experience, and some of my patients, it felt like someone had taken a belt sander to my groin for the first four weeks. There may be a burning, rash like sensation that is painful and uncomfortable for the next three to four weeks. Keep up your prescribed medications. I did have some relief with diaper rash ointment, such as Triple Paste cream. Do not apply it in or on the surgical site, and check with your physician first. Apply just to the sides of your vagina and groin area, definitely NOT between the anus and your vagina. This area is called the perineum, and the area is considered part of the wound and is still healing.

Bruising may be extensive throughout the inner thigh and abdomen. Personally and professionally, I recommend using arnica two to three times a day as needed those first four weeks. Some individuals will have bruising that will be contained to the lower abdomen; others may have bruising throughout the inner thigh as well. *For me, using arnica topically, most of my bruising was contained and disappeared completely in less than 10 days.*

I only had a small amount of bruising of my lower left abdomen, but your amount of bruising and area may be different from the next person. I believe it was the post operative application of arnica ointment and bromelain capsules that prevented the bruising from progressing into my inner thigh or further up my abdomen. Finding what works for you and keeping hydrated will also help. Proper hydration will help your blood and lymph system move the bruising out of the area. There are some folks who never bruise on the inner thigh and others just in the abdomen. We are all different and unique individuals, and our bodies heal and recover in their own enigmatic way.

Sitz Bath

The most favorable way to prevent infection in any newly opened wound area is to keep it clean. It may help if we look at sitz baths as **the most optimal** way to keep your surgical site clean and disinfected. There are some who do not like their sitz bath time. I, on the other hand, loved the sitz bath time and appreciated everything it was doing for the site. I came to describe it as my own personal mini hot tub. Keep your water mildly hot. If it is too hot, you can irritate or even scald the area and surrounding skin. Check the water with your finger before going for your dunk.

An added benefit of the sitz bath is that the warm water will help you with the sloughing of any skin during those first three to eight weeks. This includes those with shallow depth procedures too. The sitz bath is a fundamental way to keep the surgical site clean and disinfected. A small dollop of vinegar or a drop of antibacterial soap will assist in cleaning, but not irritate, your healing skin. I cannot stress enough how important a sitz bath is. Those first two to eight weeks, the sitz bath is the **best** way to keep your vagina on the healthy healing path, since you should not be scrubbing your genitals during your showers. The sitz bath felt so good, I would soak for 10 minutes rather than five to seven. I preferred it prior to a.m. dilation and p.m. dilation; the warm water seemed to make dilation easier by relaxing the pelvic floor muscles and tissue around the vaginal opening. Knowing that a sitz bath is the best way to keep the surgical site clean, I would recommend twice a day if possible!

Air it Out

The first 21 days can be arduous at times. The itching and burning sensations in your groin are not easy to work through on some days. During weeks two through six, you may consider airing out the surgical site. To do this, lay spread-eagle on your bed or with your knees apart with feet together pulled up towards your bottom in a butterfly position (Image 7).

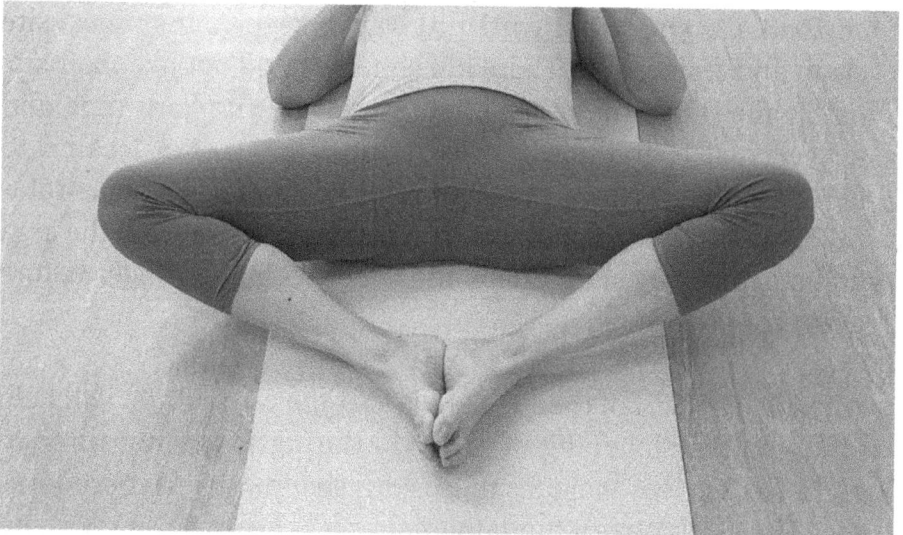

(Image 7)

Let the whole region air dry. The region is swollen, red, sore, and irritated. It is often kept in the dark and is covered, which can mean a build-up of moisture in the area. After one of your showers or a sitz bath, try just laying out on a towel to dry the area out. Allowing those legs to remain opened up will also help stretch the groin area, and you can begin to practice some massage (see massage section). Putting this into your weekly routine will help in your recovery.

Sloughing Skin

This is a tough subject for some of us. Within the first few days and weeks, the body will slough off some unnecessary skin from inside your vagina or around your vaginal opening. When this happens, the skin will look pale, yellow or gray–anything but normal flesh color–and it may hang off or slough off of the surgical site. CONSULT YOUR SURGEON! Personally, I thought my graft had fallen out; thankfully, it hadn't. Most often, it is just some dead skin that needs to be removed and is not too uncommon. In some cases patients will see their surgeon regularly those first 30 days of post-op, and they will assess and remove any dead tissue. In many cases, the removal of this unneeded tissue will make dilation easier.

Douching

To douche, or douching, means "to wash or soak." In your case, it is to wash out the inside of your vagina. The easiest place to do this is in the shower. Most surgical clinics will provide some guidelines for you prior to surgery. You can purchase your douching products at most drug stores or online. Some douches come with a premade mixture of vinegar, baking soda, or iodine. Others will just sell the container and applicator, leaving you to make your own mixture.

Be careful of the temperature when making your own mixture. Too hot and you will feel it! The inside of your vagina is very sensitive at this point. Mix two tablespoons of vinegar with water; put on the applicator, insert, and squirt. You can also do it over a toilet, but it is harder to maneuver the douche into place. Hence it is easiest to just use the shower if you can. Once you squirt the mixture internally, it will immediately come out. It is a great way to flush out any residual sloughing skin during these first six weeks.

My personal preference was two tablespoons of apple cider vinegar and one cup of warm water. Later on, I used half teaspoon soap, one tablespoon vinegar to one cup of water. Becoming familiar with douching these first three weeks will help to clear out the smell you will get that first six weeks, too. If you are doing your douche at night, not all of the liquid may drain from your vagina and may potentially dribble into your undies and bed.

The Smell

There is a fair amount of skin that once lived externally that is now learning to live internally. That tissue is not used to living inside our bodies. It will take time for our bodies to adapt. Much of the unnecessary skin will show up as sloughing discharge in your pads, with douching, or in your sitz baths. Those first six weeks, your body will slowly remove that unwanted tissue as mentioned above. It may be removed easier with regular douching.

However, the odor that is released is really smelly, I mean bad! I mean really smelly! Like YUCKY! This smell will go away generally within 3 or so weeks, although it will help you to douche on a regular basis to rinse out that smell. My surgeon described it as the "smelly sock" stage. I dubbed it the Nasty Halitosis Breath stage, which went on for 3 to 4 weeks. My partner described it as very, very stinky! That being said, whatever you experience, one of the optimal ways to move through this phase is to douche daily.

Emotions

You are not just physically healing. This procedure requires emotional healing as well. You are healing from years of being in the wrong body, experiencing dysphoria, and having an incongruous sense between body and gender. There is healing that must be done while experiencing the sensation of being in a complete and correct body. This part of your transition may be painful, not just from the surgery and wounds, but from transitioning out of a body that was not correct. Embrace the euphoric joy as well as any dysphoric grief that comes with this feeling of completeness. Like physical wounds, this takes time to heal and can be helped with a licensed therapist.

When we let go of something, there will be grief. These feelings will come up one way or another. Have a journal handy; write poetry; work on that book, or just draw your emotions with some art therapy. Whatever that may look like, give it time. Visually you see the "V" you needed, yet the region itself may not yet look like the beautiful vagina and genitals you pictured in your head. This may be overwhelming. My surgeon kept documenting it with a photo whenever I saw them. At times it was heartbreaking to know it did not look like I thought it would. Thankfully, this will change over time.

When there was necrotic skin hanging down from my new vagina, it caused me ceaseless dysphoria and personal agony thinking my graft had failed. It was beyond anything I had heard about. I was so glad I had a medical and family team that helped me through these taxing times. Knowing that you are not alone and reaching out to people for support is important.

Pads

There are moments in each individual's transition that can be extremely validating. For some trans-femmes, finding themselves at home in feminine care aisle can be one of those profound feelings, like placing the correct block into the correct hole. By week six, I was at home in that aisle of the store. By the end of the third month, I was mostly finished with full pads, and tapering to pantyliners for the next three months. Having a number of pads or panty liners handy in your purse for those first six months can be invaluable.

Emotionally, you may feel euphoria with every glance at your new genitals. With that being said, there may also be dysphoria with the sensations of being surgically pulled into a tuck for these first four to six weeks coming from the powerful sutures around the clitoris. Breathe deeply with each emotion that ebbs and flows, and recognize the first three weeks can be mentally and physically trying. Take the time to soothe your mind.

As a transgender woman, I had already gone through two transitions, one to socially transition and one to hormonally transition. With this confirmation surgery, I did not realize the depth of this procedure psychologically. For me, it was a different type of embodiment that I had not experienced before. It was a profound aspect of my transition that I would have never realized if I had not done it. It was something akin to not realizing how bad I felt until I finally felt good. It was only then that I realized how much being in the wrong body had mentally cost me every day.

On a personal note, before transitioning, I will tell you that it used to annoy me when other trans women would tell me that having bottom surgery was profound and changed their psyche. I felt like they were telling me that they were better

64

because they had gone through the surgery–like I wasn't trans enough. Being on the other side, I now know what they meant. It doesn't mean that I wasn't trans enough or that I was less of a woman because I did not have surgery, but it does change one's psyche and embodiment. It doesn't mean that I am better than other trans women–We all transition differently and have to make our own decisions about what we want and what we don't want. I have sadly heard too many stories of belittlement by gals who have gone through surgery at those who have not. Let's be kind to each other and our different journeys.

Sneezing and Coughing

Our pelvic floor is a very busy place when we sneeze or cough. When coughing or sneezing, your body is trying to eject something out of your system that it does not want., usually at high speed. I was so afraid to cough or sneeze those first three weeks. I seriously thought I would blow out a stitch. In the hospital, they will direct you to practice some deep breathing in order to stave off any problems with your lungs after surgery such as bronchitis or pneumonia. That is why it is a good idea to bring the spirometer home with you.

Continuing these exercises at home may help prevent coughing. However, there may come a time when you have to cough or sneeze while dilating. My advice is to let that dilator go; do not try to hold the dilator in during this process. If you hold your dilator in when coughing or sneezing these first six weeks, <u>it will hurt!</u> Your pelvic floor is still swollen, and it will grab hold of your dilator and can cause some serious pain. The first time I coughed while dilating the discomfort was excruciating and something I did not want to experience again, *so my advice is to just let that dilator go.*

Nerves, Tissue, and Your Inevitable Nerve Zinger

Yes, you now have your new vagina! Stop and celebrate that fact because we now have to talk about nerves. There is a bigger picture when it comes to the nerves in the surgical area. We have just had highly sensitive nerves and tissue surgically cut and relocated. Your entire genital area has been completely and elegantly remodeled. I will repeat, the healing process for this procedure takes time. Because some of this area has been cut, moved, and reattached, there will be different sensations, numb areas, and hypersensitive areas. Nerves are trying to analyze their new location, while all the surrounding tissue is trying its hardest to heal and decrease inflammation. With the relocation of these precious nerves and delicate tissue, all the body wants to do now is heal. The funny thing about nerves is, they are not like muscle or skin tissue in their healing process. Nerve healing is slower and takes longer (sometimes much longer). A nerve's healing response also comes with some electrifying results.

With all of these nerves being rearranged, your body and your brain are doing their hardest to reconnect. This reconnection will take time. Remember, some nerves that used to sit on the outside are now learning to sit on the inside or in other locations. These nerves are connected to muscles, soft tissue, and the mind. As things heal and awaken, you will inevitably get what I refer to as the Nerve Zinger. This is when a nerve sends a shooting response into that area or region. These zingers are a good sign; it means your nerves are working and trying to heal. However, the sensation is that of electricity shooting down into a nerve fiber or cluster, like you touched a live wire.

Oftentimes, you will get them when the tissue around the site is swollen and inflamed. It may remind some readers of electrolysis on a magnitude of 1000. The discomfort can and will double you over, leaving you speechless and breathless. These zingers can occur anywhere in the surgical area, but most of mine were located along a suture line. You may also have one into your clitoris, just breathe through it, and it passes just as quick as it came on. All of these weird sensations are positive manifestations of healing. I cannot stress the importance of self-massage with the use of arnica. It is THE best way to mitigate those sensations. A hot compress has shown to soothe those nerve zingers too.

There are a tremendous amount of sutures involved with this procedure. The first few weeks, if you hold your bladder too long, you will feel it into your sutures around your vulva and the mons pubis (Image 8). The vulva is made up of the external portions of the clitoris, labia majora, and the vaginal opening. This sensation will later condense to the mons pubis and clitoris in the coming months. You may actually have some sutures on the inner portion of the graft in your vagina as well. The swelling around the mons pubis and vulva will cause some discomfort in the sutures around the area during those first few weeks too. Follow your doctor's medication recommendations, and use ice in the initial stages of your recovery followed by hot compresses later on.

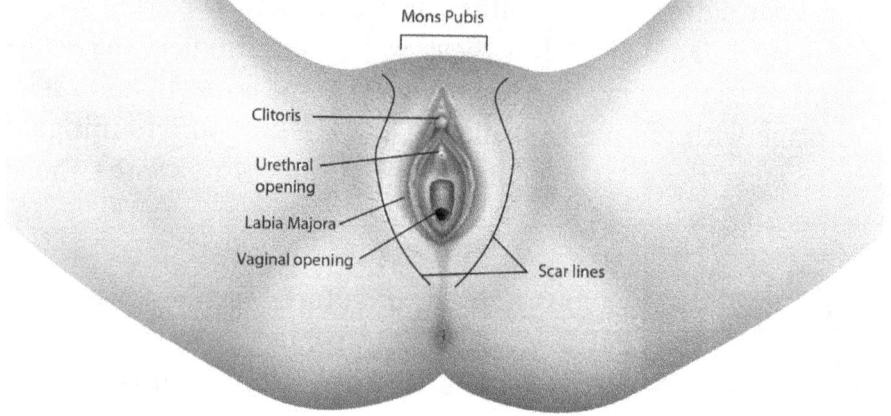

Mons Pubis

Clitoris

Urethral opening

Labia Majora

Vaginal opening

Scar lines

(Image 8)

Knowing that these nerves have been reorganized and will be trying to bring normalcy to the area may help you. There is one thing that will really help: massage. In the next chapter I have given a few massage techniques that will promote blood flow into the surgical site. These simple massage strokes around the surgical region promotes blood flow, decreases recovery time and hastens healing.

Numb Skin Patches

There is so much going on those first few weeks. It may be hard to recognize that you may have some small patches of numb skin or tissue. Within the first few weeks, I noticed that I had an area of skin that was still numb. As time passed, the region became smaller and very localized. Nerves take time to regenerate and reconnect. I have had a few patients with whom I saw nerve regeneration take one to two years. It takes time and patience.

Self-massage therapy will help tremendously. In the acupuncture field, some of us are taught a number of techniques to stimulate nerves and reduce numb patches of tissue. If you find you have numb areas that are not recovering as you would like, seek out the help of a professional acupuncturist.

One friend who was eight months out from her surgery had asked me about how to help a small numb patch on their skin. Because of where she was at in her post-op recovery (8 months) I recommended self massage and a vibrator to stimulate the tissue. Basic vibration encourages the nerve tissue to regenerate by stimulating the nerve. This will help the brain to connect back with those particular nerves. I've seen nerves recover in two different aspects of my professional career. As a professional massage therapist I helped a number of patients regain their nerve sensation through regular, consistent massage therapy, stretching and exercise. As an acupuncturist, there are even more tools that can help those with postoperative nerve issues. While you are probably not trained to do acupuncture, I will cover how to do acupressure which will also help in your healing.

Many of your nerves are for tactile sensation; it takes time to relearn things as a nerve. Learning self-massage is one of your best bets to help your recovery progress forward. Personally and professionally, I NEVER recommend the use of a vibrator to assist with numb patches of tissue within the first eight weeks; self-massage is best during that time frame. During those first eight weeks, your nerves need to calm down before applying any extra stimulation, such as vibrations.

In the realm of acupuncture, there is a technique we are taught in graduate school on the many uses of moxibustion or moxa ("MAAH-suh") for short. Moxa is made out of the herb mugwort. Mugwort orally benefits digestive problems and irregular menstruation among a few other things. Moxibustion we use to burn in various techniques is made from the pollen of the Mugwort plant. Moxibustion goes back a few thousand years as a medical therapy in acupuncture. One technique is to roll small balls of moxa and place them on top of an acupuncture needle, and burn them. This particular action nourishes the body's energy in a very specific way.

There are a few other direct techniques that require professional hands. Seeing an acupuncturist within the first 6 weeks will have profound effects on speeding your recovery and decreasing your pain. As for using moxa on nerves or numb skin it should be utilized **after** the eight week mark. If you are seeking out an acupuncturist for care, ask them if they have worked on postoperative nerve damage. Probe them to see if they are an LGBTQIA ally. Ask if they are familiar with indirect and direct moxa techniques. You will be asking this person to perform work on you in a very personal and sensitive area. Please understand that not all acupuncturists are comfortable with this technique or working in that particular area, so make sure you find someone who is supportive and knowledgeable.

There may be the possibility of sutured or caught skin nerves. It is not that common. However, if it does happen, it is not pleasant! Because there are over 150 sutures involved in this procedure, there are a lot of opportunities for these surface nerves to be impacted. Nerves can be very small and impossible to see with the naked eye; therefore sometimes they get directly impacted by a particular suture. When a superficial skin nerve is sutured it will hurt under the skin or around the sutured area. If the issue persists, it will be very helpful to consult your medical practitioner. Please know that it will take up to a year to completely heal and recover from a full depth surgery. Have patience; check-in with your physical therapist, and consult the Scar Tissue section in .

Chapter 4

Pain Management

Pain management is in your hands. Use your pain meds as needed, but know that there is danger of becoming addicted to them as well. The use of a spinal block has shown to reduce the abuse of opioids, which is an added benefit if your surgeon chooses to do one. There may come a time in these first 12 weeks where a stitch, suture, or the physical pain of pooling blood into your pelvic floor is too much. Being attentive to any opioid consumption is vital. Surprisingly, the common recommendation of tylenol and regular anti-inflammatories or NSAIDs (non steroidal anti-inflammatory) work amazingly well. Keep your opioid for those moments and times when your anti-inflammatories are not doing the job.

Personal Advice: At one point, the pain of one particular suture near my clitoris was so excruciating that I needed to break through the pain. I was exhausted. When we are in pain, we do not heal as well or as swiftly. So, knowing when to use your opioid medication is important, especially during this time period, as we start to become more mobile, and internal stitches begin to move and tug. Pain is often subjectively measured on a scale from one to 10. I use the word "subjective" because pain is different for everyone. An eight on a pain level to me may be a five to others. Most times, tylenol and ibuprofen do a great job, but when they do not work, using an opioid to BREAK THROUGH the pain will pay off. Don't be the tough girl and try to work through it without pain medication—You will heal better and more quickly by controlling your pain.

Dilation: Your Physical Therapy

Let's get some things clear; your pelvic floor is in nearly continuous use all day long. The pelvic floor is a support structure for your whole body. The pelvic floor wants to pinch or close off your new vagina. The body wants to close holes. Period! This particular muscle group has an inherent nature to control posture, so generally, all the pelvic muscles are always turned on. So when you begin to dilate, learning to release your pelvic floor and loosening it up with some pelvic floor stretches will help ease the discomfort. You can find those stretches in the Pre-op Preparation Stretching section in Chapter 1. With all the recent renovation done in this area, when you dilate there might be pulling on your vulva and/or on your clitoris. The size area between an AMAB pelvis and an AFAB pelvis is physiologically smaller, and your vagina was squeezed into a space between your bladder and your bowel (Image 9). This reduced space may lead to some struggle with dilation.

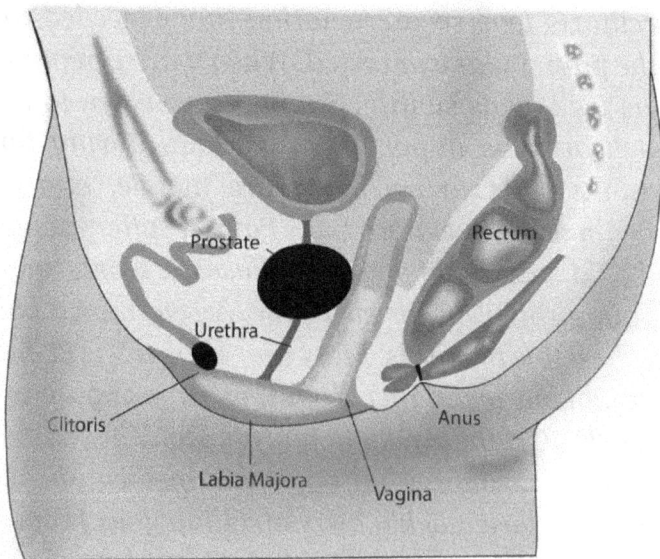

(Image 9)

Dilation is your physical therapy. Dilation has two facets, one to help the diameter of your vagina and the second is depth. You must be diligent, remain calm, breathe, and take a break if needed. We are dealing with very delicate tissue. You must go slow, finding your own pace. During these first 12 weeks, you should **not** stop dilating. It does get much easier and less painful after four months. But these four months can be grueling.

Let's cover a few things that can help you. First, prior to your dilation session, go to the bathroom. Evacuating your bladder and your bowels prior to dilation will help with discomfort. As you can see from image 9, the dilator will be pressing the bladder and the bowel when you dilate. Second, the dilator should be angled up toward your belly button. Thirdly, lube up. Those first few weeks of dilating finding the right amount of lube is messy but important. Having a towel or disposable Chux pad underneath you will prevent lube from getting on everything and will allow you to use extra lube, which is great when first beginning.

Yes it can become more messy, but we are learning, and at times learning can be messy. There can be an increase of pain when using too little lubricant. So lube up that dilator, gently insert a little and take it out. Work the dilator slowly in, and breathe deeply as you need to. At times you may have to push and breath through the pain. Once again, it is delicate skin that has just had surgery upon it. Be gentle. I have read countless times that issues arise if not enough lube is used. Your dilator can get stuck, which is unpleasant. If this happens, you want to slowly wiggle it from side to side until you get it loose. Turning your dilator until it comes loose is a good method too. If worse comes to worse, just take a finger and slide it right next to the dilator to bring some air into the area.

When I first considered this surgery, I had heard about "dilation stations" from one gal. Then I heard it from a few others. Having a calm, comfortable setting is important, as is keeping everything you need for dilation in one place. This will become your dilation station. Your body placement for dilation is important. Laying on your back is best; do NOT prop your torso up with pillows. Your arms will likely get tired from holding the dilator in place—and sometimes your arms just aren't long enough to comfortably do it.

Another option is to use the heels of your feet to hold it in place. However, if you use your heels to hold the dilator in, you can activate your pelvic floor, which may make it harder to dilate. Test this out, and see how your body responds. It may be easy for some of you to drop into a butterfly position with your legs opened and your feet together, and this is one of the reasons why focusing on stretching techniques before surgery is important. Trans women have been very resourceful at finding other ways to comfortably dilate. Some lay on a towel and pull the towel up (think of a loin cloth) over the dilator to hold it in place. Find what works for you, and consult your physical therapist because you will be spending a lot of time dilating, and you don't want the process to be miserable because you aren't comfortable.

We need to create depth and width, yet we need to hold the dilator in for 15 to 20 minutes. Finding what works for you will be on the top of your agenda. I had been encouraged by other trans women to use a long towel and use the towel to hold the dilator in. However, the physical therapist did make me aware that this is not the best angle, but for some of us, it works. Once again, the dilator should be angled up toward the belly button. If it is angled toward the colon, you may pass some gas or irritate your colon by pressing against it through the vaginal wall. Finding a position where it hurts the least takes time. I will tell you it does become easier. Previously I have mentioned some pre-dilation stretches in Chapter 1. During these first 6 weeks keep these stretches simple and unforced. This means just lean into the stretches, and do not feel like you should push hard into these basic stretches. You can and will hurt yourself if you are overly aggressive with your time while in the stretch itself.

While dilating you do not ever want to apply too much excess pressure! Applying enough pressure to keep the dilator in, do not try to drive a hole through our new vagina. You may rupture the back of your vagina, which would require another surgery to fix. Your primary goal is to keep the vagina open. I cannot stress enough the importance of releasing the pelvic floor during the dilation process. You want to feel the pelvis exhale downwards or outwards. The action of releasing a bowel movement is one way of releasing the pelvic floor. Doing this during dilation takes practice, time, and a little relaxation. If your physical therapist suggests any particular lube, get it. Try it out, and find what works for you. *I tried one and found another on the list that worked better and have used it ever since.*

Personally, those first three weeks, I did not go wild with dilation. I used the smallest dilator for three weeks. Despite the strong sutures, you do not want to make tears in your graft. Your focus is just to not allow your vaginal cavity to close. I've known a few women that tore or ripped some of the graft. It was not pleasant, and some had to go in for secondary surgery. I didn't go up a dilator size until the 22nd day. Only when I was certain that the sutures had healed up from my medical team did I move up a size or pressure.

Unfortunately that incremental different size does hurt, but you are making progress, I promise. Find your rhythm or pace; apply pressure for a minute or 30 seconds, and then stop applying pressure for 30 seconds and try to build up from there. As I mentioned earlier, your new vagina is still a healing surgical site during the first six weeks. The tissue is extremely delicate and has a fundamental sensitivity. Breathing and having a mindful touch will help your recovery.

One other important facet during your dilation times is distraction. If you are constantly looking at the clock, time will often move slower. Set your timer, and groove into your distraction. This is a great time to explore an audio book or to watch a movie. Finding a few different distractions will help you down the road. These simple diversions will make the time go by faster. Here are some ideas that may help:

Set your dilation timer, but do not look at the time!

- Explore audio books.

- Watch a movie.

- Watch funny videos on YouTube.

- Light gaming.

- Virtual reality device.

- Music.

- Talking with your partner.

Finding whatever type of distractions works for you is most important. I had a patient get a virtual reality device, and that was a game changer for them. But I am very aware that not all of us have the ability to afford a VR device. If you can borrow one, it may help. Up to this point I had never considered it, but I thought it would be applicable here. I did end up borrowing a VR device during this time frame, and it was incredibly helpful. This time is for you and you only. Find your symphony, your rock band, your game, and you choose the tempo.

*Sound Medicine: As mentioned previously, it is best **not to miss any sessions of dilation**! Here is the medical reason behind that. The natural instinct of the body is to close things, such as holes, a wound or a newly formed cavity, like our new vagina. This is a hard pill to swallow. Those first few weeks, the body naturally wants to, and will try to, close the newly formed vaginal opening. Dilation prevents this from happening. The down side, if you do not dilate regularly is that you can lose vaginal depth and width quickly these first 8 weeks.*

More Advice: The second part of the advice is keep the dilator in for an extra three to five minutes. UGH, I know it will hurt. If you dilate for 15 minutes, just adding on an extra three to five minutes does go a long way in the development of our vagina, but it is not necessary.

*Simple Recommendation: This information comes directly from my friend Jessica. At the end of week two, I consulted her about lube, and she said, "Once you find the one you like, **buy a ton of it!**" These next six months, you will go through a whole bunch of lube. I tried three different kinds and settled on Slippery Stuff. And I bought a three-pack on amazon.*

Good Suggestion: Another valuable suggestion came from a lady who had her surgery in the Philadelphia area. She said "Whatever you do, DO NOT miss ONE dilation session!" That is hard to hear these first eight weeks, I know. It pays off in another eight weeks, when your pelvic floor inflammation subsides and the risk of stenosis or narrowing is decreased. If you do miss a dilation time these first eight weeks, there is the potential of losing some depth.

Lidocaine

Ask for lidocaine, PERIOD! I really wish this was part of the take-home medication. Dilation hurts those six to 12 weeks and particularly if you have any granulation (see below). Lidocaine applied five minutes before your daily dilation routine will ease that initial penetration discomfort and soothe some of the pelvic floor discomfort. *I am also here to reassure you that with time dilation does become easier and much less uncomfortable.*

Granulation

What is granulation? This is just one form of healing your body has but it results in a grainy type of tissue that is red and irritated. Granulation typically occurs at the vaginal opening and is caused from the repeated stretching which causes micro-tears of the tissue. The sensation feels like grains of sand at the opening of your vagina. Granulation can appear in different areas as well over the course of the next few weeks.

This is a great time to make an appointment to see your physician, as they can easily remove any affected tissue through the painless application of silver nitrate. It does really make a difference. Granulation can happen from two to 12 weeks post-op. If you cannot see your physician, applying some lidocaine prior to dilation will ease some of the symptoms. Add more lube to the opening of your vagina and to your dilator. Over time, the body will heal the area.

Any Ongoing Discomfort

You may have ongoing pelvic floor pain. I did, as did some of my patients. It took a few visits to my physical therapist to recognize that one of my hip rotators was sore and/or tight. Your hip rotators rotate your legs inward and outward. After a few exercises working on my leg rotators, it decreased. Don't be afraid to talk to your doctor or physical therapist about any particular problems you are experiencing while dilated. A good pelvic floor specialist should be able to provide some exercises that will provide relief as well.

Personal thoughts: In moving up a size in your dilators, one way to breakthrough some discomfort is to slowly increase to a larger/wider dilator during the last five minutes of your dilation time. Start with your smallest dilator, and then those last few minutes of dilation, go for the next size up. Slowly work up to the larger dilator, and follow your physician's or physical therapist's advice.

Different Dilators

Around week four, it was recommended to me by my physical therapist to find a more comfortable dilator. The dilators I was given were designed by Dr. Marci Bowers and are made from hard plastic. They are each nine inches long, and they step up incrementally in diameter from 1 ⅛", 1 ¼", 1 ⅜" and 1 ½" (Image 10).

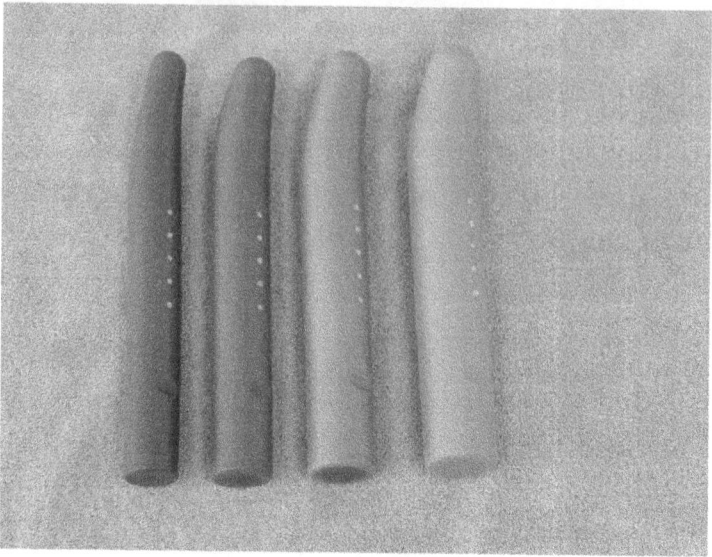

(Image 10)

At this point, I was having some small problems with dilating, and my physical therapist recommended a few other options; that is when I landed on the dilators by Intimate Rose. The photo provided is of their 1 ¼" and 1 ½" diameter sizes. (Image 11).

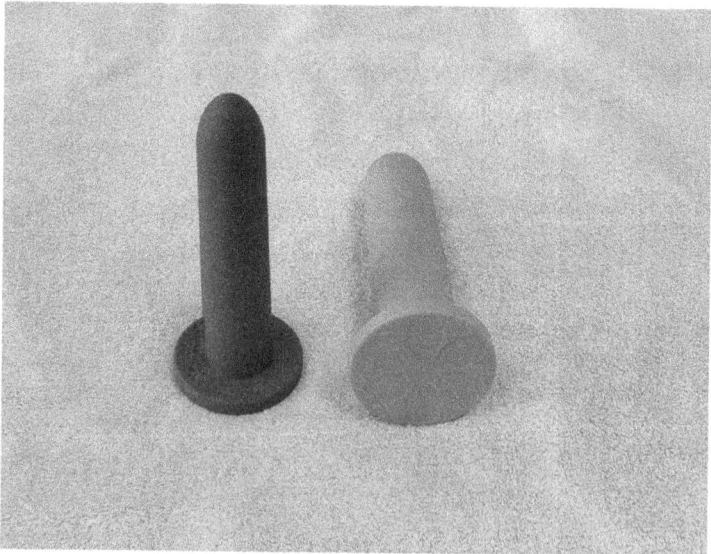

(Image 11)

These dilators are made from silicone and are therefore softer. They come in the same widths but are shorter. Holding them in can be done with a towel more easily and, as a bonus, they also fit into a strap-on nicely. Eventually, I went back to using the hard plastic ones because they are longer and easier to hold in place, but feel free to try different options. Please check with your surgeon and physical therapist to make sure whatever you are deciding on will work. I encourage you to do your own research. You may actually find something else that works. This is just a guide to help you heal and recover happily.

Dilator Preparation

I've heard of folks chilling or cooling their dilators prior to use. Personally, I soaked my dilators in a pitcher of hot tap water prior to use. My professional thought is that muscles and soft tissue like heat, despite the natural inflammation of the area. Often, muscles will soften up when heat is applied. You will want your sore and inflamed pelvic floor muscles to be relaxed. This is anecdotal, but it helped me. After eight weeks, I stopped soaking my dilators in hot water and just cleaned them and used them at room temperature. But your renovated genitals are swollen and hurt when dilating, so finding what works for you is important. Remember to wash your dilators after every use.

Serious consideration: I know a few folks who don't want to or do not have penetrative sex, so depth and width is not a concern. So staying with a smaller dilator is cool too. No peer pressure from me.

Personal advice: I tried to dilate for 30 minutes those first two weeks of dilation. Oh It hurt more, and I was physically exhausted from the pain. For me, I found 20 minutes seemed to be a good medium. My physical therapist clarified things when I came in with consistent pelvic floor pain at the end of week.

She suggested when we dilate three times a day, the pelvic floor becomes inflamed. So with a longer dilation session, the surrounding tissue of my vagina (the pelvic floor) was in fact being inflamed from regular dilation. I tapered down to 20 minutes, and the result was much better.

Douching

Douching your vagina takes practice and time. You might make some mistakes along the way, but if you practice it enough, it becomes second nature. Keep an eye on your water temperature! Do not make it too hot, or it will hurt you. By the 10 to 15 week point, you will be a pro. I sometimes would do a quick douche after each dilation session to both rinse myself out and to practice; it paid off. For me, douching tapered off around week 12 to once or twice a week rather than daily.

It is important to douche regularly with a little apple cider vinegar about once a week. Do not be surprised in the first six weeks when you will see sloughing skin come out of your vagina and or a stitch. Be concerned if you see excessive or consistent bleeding. You will be douching for the rest of your life because our vaginas do not produce natural secretions, so getting good at it will make your life easier.

Padsicles

A padsicle is a regular pad with some Aloe Vera and bacitracin put on before you wear it *(Image 12)*. You can also freeze them to further assist with the healing. The Aloe soothes suture lines and irritated skin. Bacitracin is an antibacterial ointment to keep the site moist and prevent infection. I came up with my own vaginoplasty padsicle recipe, and I ran it by my surgeon;

she approved it. However, please consult your own medical professionals.

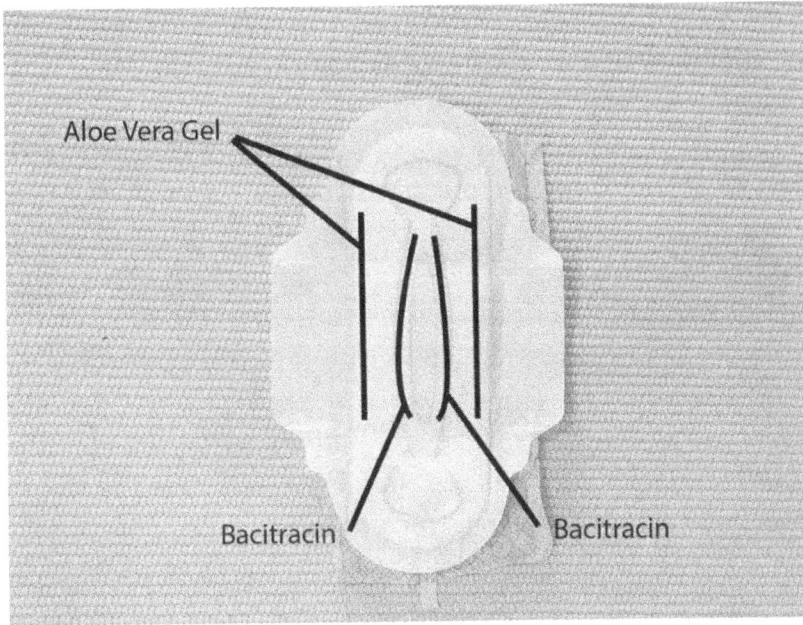

(Image 12)

Padsicle Supplies: (Consult your surgeon or physician)

- One large overnight pad.

- Open one pad, but do not remove it from the sticky backing.

- Apply Aloe Vera to the pad (a nice circle around the edge of the pad.) I used extra Aloe those first few weeks because of a rash and burning sensation.

- Apply bacitracin to the center of the pad.

- Fold back up and place in a freezer bag or container, or place in your undies right away.

When you need a fresh pad placed in your underwear, you will have a nice soothing sensation on your stellar new genitals.

Personal Note: I made about three to four for each day, and I always ended up with a few for the following day. The Aloe Vera with the Bacitracin was amazing for the recovery of the surgical site, and the Aloe is very soothing to the skin.

Friend's Advice: One friend found the padsicles to be too moist or wet at first. Finding the correct amount to apply to your pad is up to you. I found the extra Aloe Vera to soothe the surgical site, but use whatever works for you.

The Donut Cushion

Many, if not all of us, are encouraged to purchase or borrow a donut cushion. You will be having or have just had reconstructive surgery on and around your pelvic floor. Either shallow or full-depth procedure, our pelvic floor has been modified along with our genitals. You will not want to put direct pressure on that area for a while. In theory, donut cushions prevent your genital area from direct weight bearing when you sit—and they do for the most part. However, when we sit for too long, blood will follow gravity and will pool into the muscles of our pelvic floor, whether you are sitting on a donut or not. Since you just had surgery down there, there will be swelling, and skin will become tight and stretched due to the fluid build-up. Sometimes the donut cushion backfires and creates more fluid build-up, and therefore, more pressure on the skin of this very sensitive area due to its circular nature.

If you must sit and are using the pillow, make sure you can lay down sometimes and/or are moving around regularly. If you have sat throughout the day, you may actually find it harder to dilate just from blood pooling into the pelvic floor and swelling of the surgical site. Expect to use a cushion for 11 to 12 weeks. Around week 11, you will start to feel better about sitting. That being said, do what is comfortable for you.

As a final note on cushions, many people find that using a neck cushion is actually more comfortable than a donut cushion. Sitting on the neck cushion can allow for more blood to flow into and out of the area, rather than preventing blood flow from leaving the area. Please choose whichever cushion you find most comfortable.

Hot Compress

It is suggested to place a hot compress over the surgical site to ease tension, pain, and swelling–but only after the initial swelling of week one or two has gone down. It will be a very effective antidote when it comes to the nerve zingers mentioned earlier. Oftentimes, tap water was not hot enough, so you may want to use warmer water by heating it up in a kettle or on the stove. If you use this method, be VERY careful it is not too hot. Pour the warmed water onto a washcloth, ring out with tongs, and then wrap the wet washcloth into another dry towel (Image 13) .

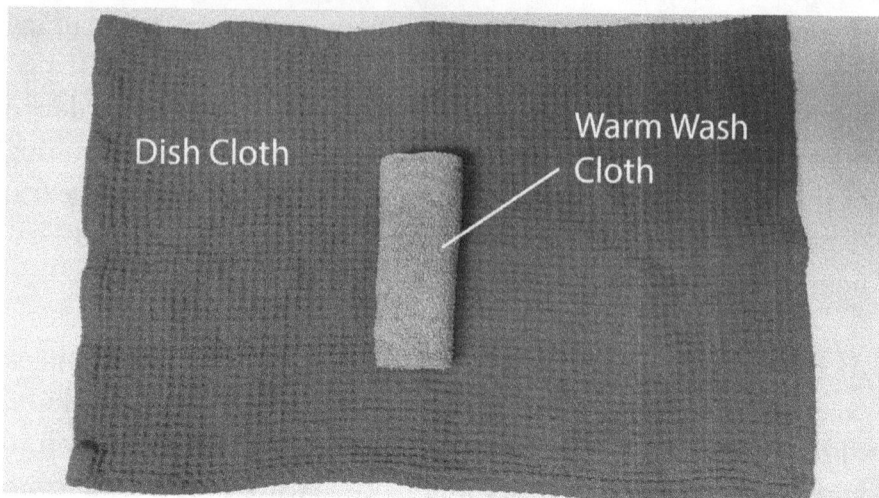
(Image 13)

I found that wrapping the washcloth in a kitchen towel worked well as it was thin enough to let the heat penetrate to my skin. Apply to mons pubis, vulva, and labia. You may be surprised at how good it feels. You may also find some other options on the interweb.

Discharge and Menstrual Pads

Let me get to some serious stuff. **If you have excessive bleeding that fills your pad repeatedly from end to end, go to the ER or contact your surgeon immediately.** This is most likely to happen within the first 21 days. Once the rabbit trick of pulling 15 feet out, you will have light, bloody discharge for the next six weeks.

In your pads, you will also find a stitch or two and some dead skin. Often, the bloody discharge will follow the suture lines. Those first six weeks, the discharge is regular, consistent, and smelly. It will taper off over the next 12 weeks. You will also see skin sloughing in your pads these first four weeks. (Feel free to refer to the Nourishing Nuggets section at the end of chapter 4.)

Keeping an eye on your discharge is important. You are the primary individual who is overseeing the surgical site. If you suspect too much bleeding, contact your physician. Too much blood may be a serious issue and may need immediate medical attention. You will want to start off with the thick and large overnight pads these first three weeks. Get long or extra long, as they will give you the best coverage.

Sleep is an incredible part of your healing. During the hours that we sleep our bodies use the parasympathetic nervous system to repair and care for you. Put in a fresh overnight pad or padsicle for the night. You can also use adult diapers such as Depends. Do not be overly surprised if you find blood on your sheets. Your pad will be mildly full by the morning, a nice warm morning sitz bath will help clean the area.

Around the end of week three, most of your bleeding will have come slowly to an end, if not sooner. This should prompt you to change to a thinner pad. You will still want to have those overnight pads for the next three week stint, but during the day you can decrease to a thinner pad. You can continue using the padsicles to ease sutures and heal skin tissue. I have known some individuals who went down to a very thin small pantiliner. If you move to a smaller one too soon, they may prove to be too small and you may stain your undies. You may need to wait until after 10 to 12 weeks. Expect to get blood on your underwear– Pads do not give perfect coverage. This is why most of us buy underwear that we end up throwing out after this period.

I have had a few individuals develop rashes from the pads with wings and/or from the adhesive on the wings. Vaseline or Triple Paste for diaper rash are good products to add to your supplies and will help with pad irritation. Play around with whatever pad works best for you. Between week six and eight, you will know what pad is good for you but I have had a few patients that needed to change to a more natural pad. There are less chemicals and detergents in the more natural pads and have helped some to decrease the irritation of constantly wearing a pad for three months. They are more expensive but they will go a long way in a healthy recovery if you find that your genitals are sensitive to the chemicals in normal pads. By the end or the third or fourth month, the cotton lining in your underwear will absorb any moisture that may gather in the area.

Chapter 5

Massage, Acupressure & Reflexology

Weeks One through Three

The amazing benefits of massage go back thousands of years. In the last few hundred years, there have been detailed improvements and expansion of its beneficial modalites. There are a good number of modalities such as: deep tissue, Swedish, hot stone, lymph drainage, Shiatsu or acupressure, trigger point, reflexology, and many more. For your particular case, we will be covering Swedish massage strokes, acupressure, and reflexology. These three therapeutic modalities will be very beneficial with lasting effects. I professionally would also recommend a few Lymphatic Drainage sessions from a licensed professional trained in Manual Lymphatic Drainage. Now for a brief anatomy lesson.

There are a variety of support systems within the human body. There is the musculoskeletal system, the cardiovascular system, the nervous system, both parasympathetic (rest and digest) and sympathetic (fight or flight). In your healing process, both of these last two nervous systems have a vital aspect in your healing. Two other systems are the lymphatic system and immune system. These various systems are working to maintain a system-wide homeostasis. The two physical systems you will be working on during this chapter will be the musculoskeletal system and the lymphatic system. The musculoskeletal system pertains to the locomotion of our bodies; this includes muscles, joints, bones, and connective tissue. Connective tissue is extensive and is in nearly every nook and cranny of your body. Within the vast musculoskeletal complex, all of these other numerous systems are contained. When the system experiences trauma, psychologically or physically, there are a variety of systemic responses. Going forward, I will only be focusing on how physical trauma affects the body. I will leave the psychological trauma to licensed professionals.

On a personal and professional note; in this and any forthcoming chapters, when I am referring to trauma, it is pertaining to the invasive surgical inflammatory trauma, not to the psycho-emotional trauma of having the incorrect body.

Fascinatingly, if there is trauma to the body such as surgical trauma, the body and the surrounding tissues will remember it. There are great tools to move this mentally and physically sensory memory. Physically, when trauma occurs, your soft tissues such as muscles, fascia, and connective tissues get inflamed. These tissues remember it. The body will swell in that region, and white blood cells are sent into the area.

One of the greatest ways to break through physical surgical trauma is with gentle, compassionate massage therapy. One important aspect of massage therapy is blood flow, which helps move toxins and trauma through the lymph system. This lymph system has an inert connection to your body's immunity. This system helps with fluid levels and defends the body from infection. Light massage, basic movement, and stretches will move blood and toxins through this particular system.

Where is your lymph system? It is located throughout your body with a majority of it in your inner thighs, abdomen, armpits, neck, and chest (Image 14).

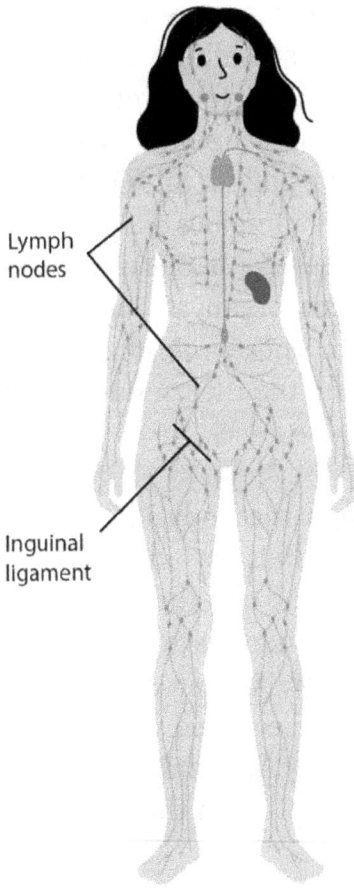

(Image 14)

How can you assist it in your healing process? By gentle, light-pressure massage, movement, and stretching. This will help with post-op swelling and excess fluid build-up. It also helps our body fight any potential infection.

Besides massage techniques, you will also be given a few acupressure points throughout this book. The acupoints systems work with a completely different type of medical system. In acupressure and acupuncture, the theories can be vast and differ greatly from Western medical practices. As a practitioner of Traditional Chinese Medicine, which has been in use for 3,000 years, there are a few components we work with. One integral aspect is something known as Qi (pronounced "Chee"); this Qi resides in all forms of life. Qi traverses the body with well over 300-plus acupoints. The terms "meridian" or "channel" pertain to the path of this Qi. In some cases, there are western anatomical organ names associated with some of these channels, as you will see later in this chapter. The older channels do not have a Western organ associated with them, but the newer channels will. These meridians have been used for thousands of years, and the theories associated with them have multiplied with time.

This Qi moves through the body in a coordinated effort in a variety of these channels or meridians. These energetic pathways are in every limb and throughout the front, back, and sides of the body. These channels work to bring harmony to your body and its own Qi flow. They do this in beautiful ways; these paths of Qi have been equated in textbooks to rivers and streams. If a river breaks the bank, flooding occurs, often into areas that were not prepared for that much water.

These rivers of Qi work to carry Qi throughout the body to harmonize your body, mind, and spirit. If these energetic channels become impaired psychologically and physically it can prevent Qi from moving smoothly throughout your body. These meridians strive to maintain the best possible harmony under all circumstances. In your particular case, there are a few channels that we interrupted during this procedure, and you can help bridge those interruptions with some basic acupressure points. If you have the means, this is where a skilled acupuncturist can tap into the medicine within you to make profound progress.

We can make profound changes with touch, too. The result of this surgery will leave the surrounding skin and tissues swollen.

The ideal way to move the inflammation out of the area and increase healing, is with self-massage. Massage will be helpful in moving the build-up of fluid in your groin, lower abdomen, and inner thighs. For the first 21 days, your self-massage should be light and gentle. Learning to perform a massage on specific regions will help in reducing your pain. The pressure of your self-massage during this time should be no more than one pound of pressure, or the <u>weight of one apple or one orange</u>.

There is empowerment in performing self-massage; you will be able to feel surgical tension leave with each and every massage stroke. The first seven days, the inner thigh and abdomen areas will be swollen and very sensitive. At this point, your body will not respond well to excess massage pressure, the lighter and gentler the better, like applying moisturizer. In fact, you might just glide your hand along your skin at first, depending on how sore you are.

If you have someone you trust and willing to help you with massage, have them read through this entire section. A skilled masseuse will check in often to see how the pressure is for you. Please take this into consideration when receiving a massage from someone else during these first six to 12 weeks. Also take into consideration that you will want to cover up your vag with a clean towel to lay upon in addition to some undies.

Personal Note: By the end of the 10th day post-op, dilation was already beyond tender, even with the prescribed medication. So 15 minutes prior to the evening dilation session, I lay down and began gently massaging my inner thighs. Within the first massage strokes, I could feel a majority of my pain just dissolve. The inner thighs held so much traumatic memory from surgery that once I massaged it, my vaginal pain went away completely.

Massage Therapy Supplies

- A box of gloves for massage the first six weeks

- Arnica or Arnicare ointment or gel

- Organic grape seed oil for massage or a massage oil of choice. Avoid those massage oils with scents added.

- Chux pads

- Reusable ice pack (Relief Pack works great)

- Washcloths for hot compress and a clean towel to wrap hot compress into.

IMPORTANT

To maintain a healthy surgical site, latex, nitrile, or vinyl **gloves are REQUIRED for the first eight weeks.** This is to keep the surgical site clean and disinfected.

Massage Therapy Week Two to Three:

Position yourself on your back with legs in butterfly position (knees open bottom of feet together) or with feet flat and your knees bent.

1) These first 21 days, you can just use an Arnica ointment. I liked to mix it with a little grape seed oil, but a massage oil of your choice will work, too. Apply arnica to gloved hands, or dab a little directly on the desired region. Arnica is tremendously helpful with bruising and

swelling, so reapply as needed. Mix the Arnica and oil for a good massage medium.

2) Using your fingers and palms, gently and lightly glide your hands from your inner knee upward toward your groin and vagina. Your hand pressure should be the weight of one orange. Repeat five to ten times on each leg. (Image 15)

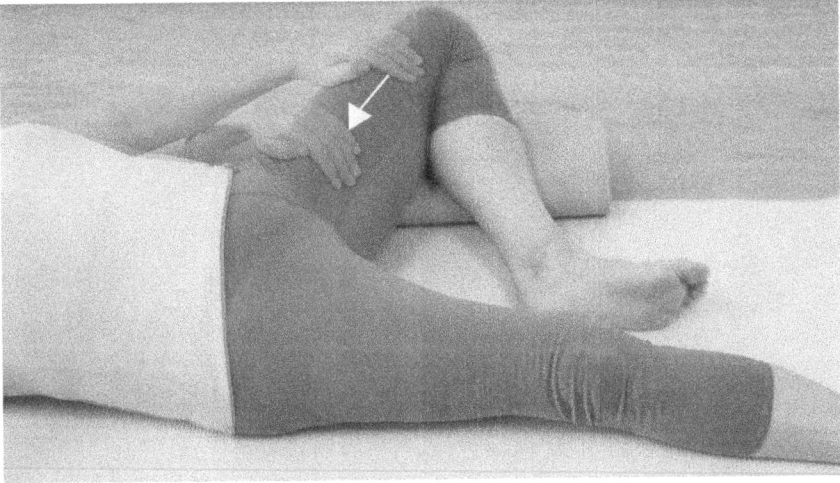

(Image 15)

3) Place your hands one on top of each other or beside each other. Then place both of your hands just below your navel (belly button) palm-down. Very gently (with the pressure of an orange), lightly perform small circular motions on the abdomen. Repeat this motion working outwards toward your large intestine nine times. Apply Arnica as needed to the lower abdomen to ease bruising and swelling. (Image 16)

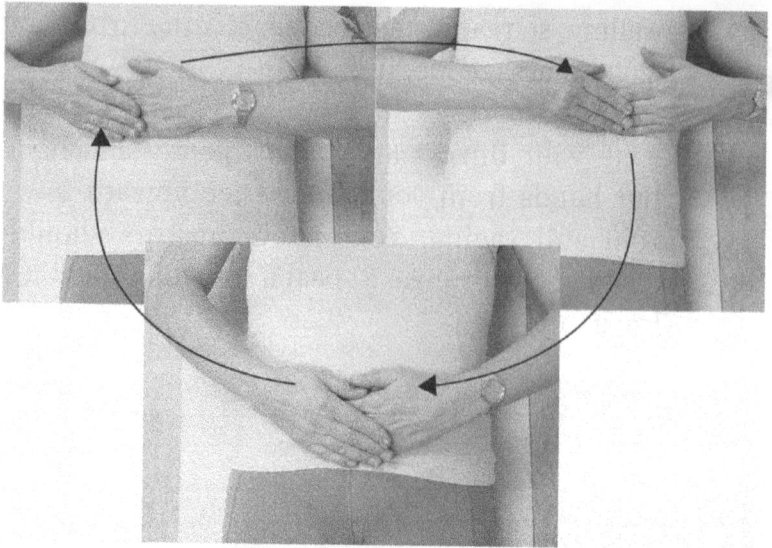

(Image 16)

4) Repeat this one to two times a day for the first three weeks.

5) The included use of Arnica ointment or gel to reduce bruising and swelling

6) Remember to use gloves up to week eight.

7) Watching your pressure during self-massage is critical! Too much pressure can lead to blood clots during these first few months. Focus on moving the surgical trauma, and keep the pressure very light and gentle.

IMPORTANT

When working on the feet and ankles, the pressure should not exceed the weight of one pound. If you are having someone else assist you for this section, keep an eye on the pressure they are using. Even if it feels good, your still healing and deep pressure mat result in a blood clot.

Reflexology

There are some specific aspects to your bodily healing and recovery represented on and around your feet. Let us look at some great reflexology regions on the feet and hands that can help you heal. When I felt the profound change in my body after the first massage, I pulled up my reflexology charts to find a way to ease more of my pain and increase the healing. In reflexology, there are a great number of areas that influence the whole body. In your case, I have given location for the genitals, intestines, heart, and lungs (Image 17 [foot] and image 17.2 [Left-hand]).

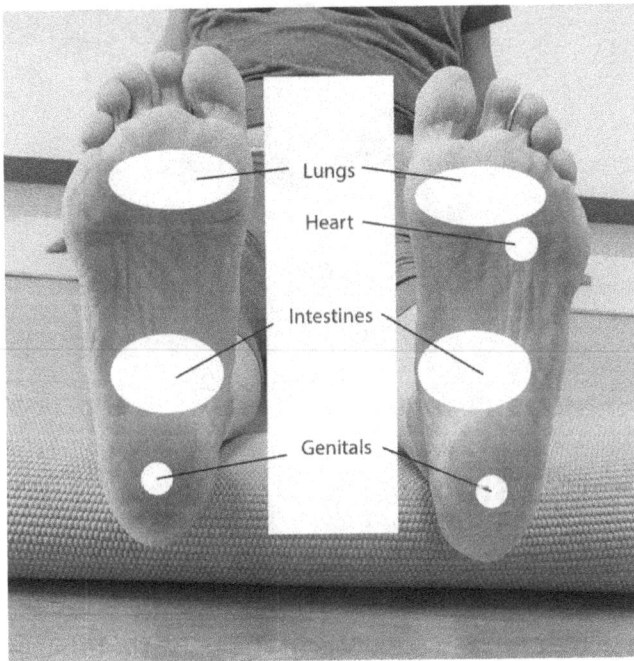

(Image 17)

The pressure should be the weight of one orange or one pound.

1) Intestinal tract region

2) Heart region

3) Lung Region

4) Genital Region

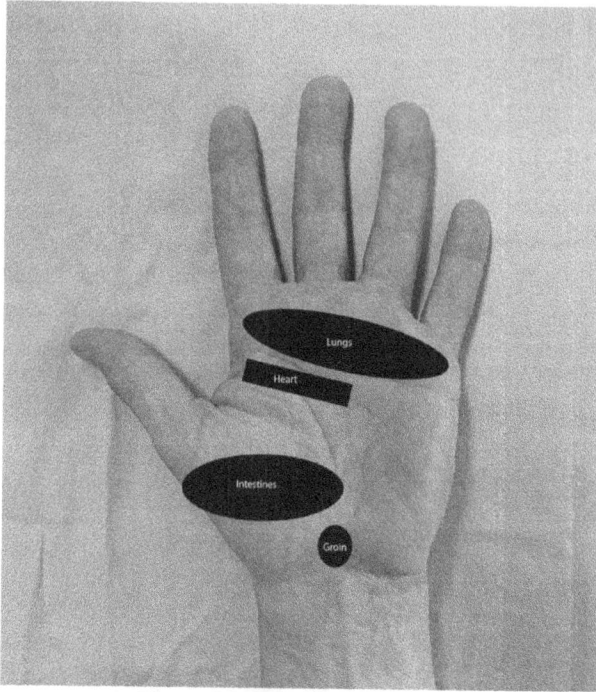

(Image 17.2)

Acupressure

In acupressure and acupuncture techniques, a channel or meridian of Qi will diverge deeper into the body to have impact on particular parts or regions of the body that the channel might be associated with. Through the use of acupressure, you have the ability to use touch to influence healing in a deeper energetic way. Similar to massage, the weight used in acupressure is one pound. Most of these will be easy to find, and there are pictures accompanying the acupressure points.

The first set of points are the easiest ones to access, and they are within reach right after the surgery. For the second set of points, you may want a friend or family member to assist you. Originally, acupoints were given formal names; in later times, they were labeled with numbers. Not only will I be giving you the formal acupoint name, but also the acupoint number. A number of these points are associated with an organ channel or meridian of Qi, as mentioned earlier. So, for instance, one acupoint will be the LU-7 (Lung - 7) point, and the formal name is called "*Broken Sequence*." This means that it is the seventh point on the Lung meridian/channel; the name *Broken Sequence* partly pertains to an aspect contained within this acupoint. There are a great number of acupoints that have influences on different parts of the body. So, let us get started on where they are located and what they affect.

Hand Acupressure

The first two acupoints are located on the wrist and hand. Despite their location, they influence two very old channels that are not associated with western organs. These two meridians run up the midline of the front and back of your body. These two meridians are known respectively as the Conception (Ren) and Governing (Du) Vessels; their Pinyin titles (Pinyin: The standard of romanized spelling for transliteration Chinese) respectively are Ren and Du.

LU-7: *Broken Sequence*, Lung 7, LU-7 is located on the wrist (Image 18).

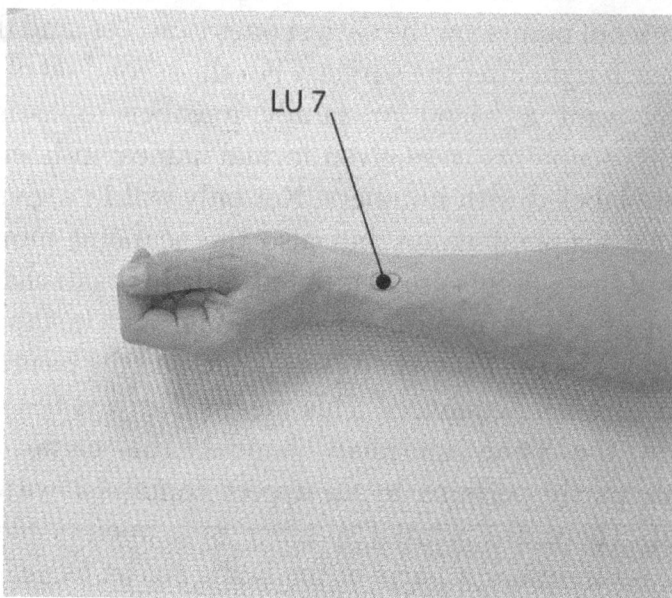

(Image 18)

Apply the pressure equivalent to the weight of an orange. Go in a circle nine times, and then repeat. Do this for two minutes on each wrist. The name is derived from the fact that its point actually breaks slightly from its sequence between LU-8 and LU-9, which runs midline up the front of the body, from our perineum to the bottom of the mouth. These points influence the center of the body and your vaginal region. That influence is directly related to providing more energy to the healing of your surgical site.

SI-3: *Back Stream*, Small Intestine-3: On the side of the hand/wrist area, apply the pressure equivalent to the weight of an orange (Image 19).

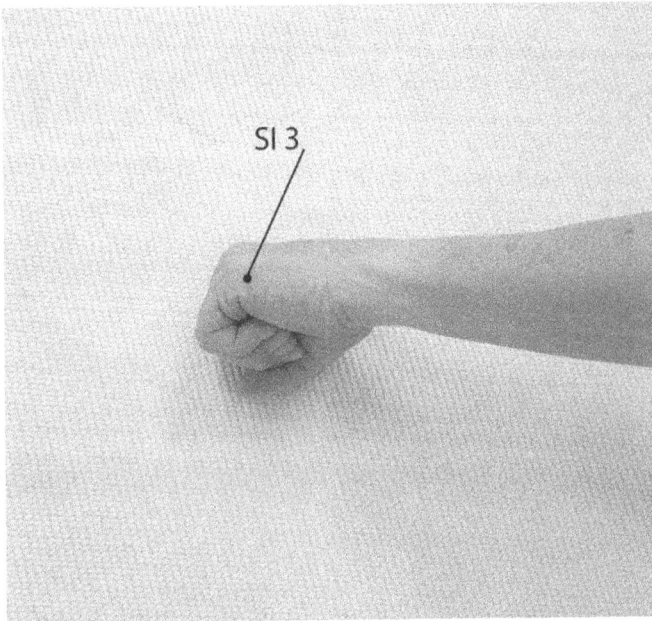

(Image 19)

Feel free to go in a circle nine times, and then repeat. Do this for two minutes on each wrist. This point influences a meridian that moves upward from the perineum along the midline of the body up the spine over the head to the roof of your mouth. This point helps the rectum, the spine, and the vaginal area.

Head and Body Acupressure

Du-20: *Hundred Meetings*, Du Mai-20: This point is located on the top of the head (Image 20).

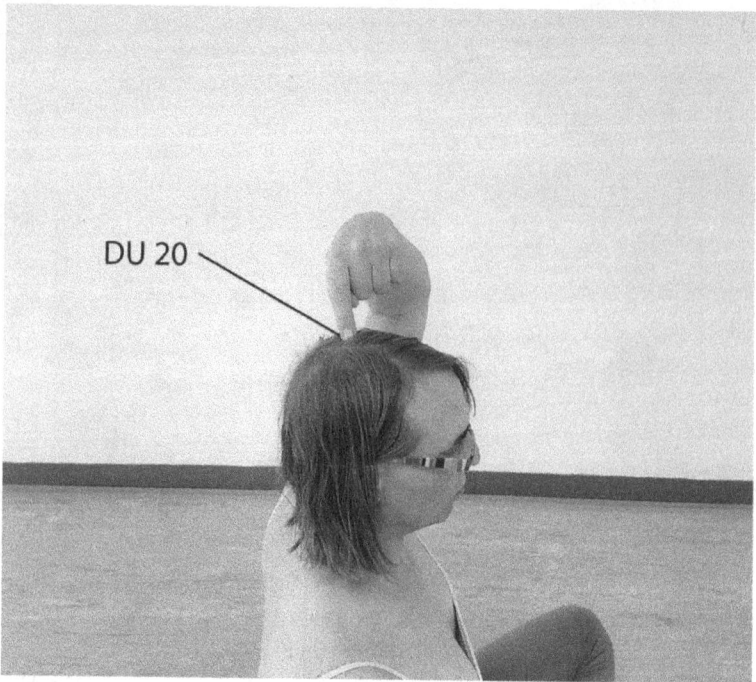

(Image 20)

It is a mirror point for our neo-vagina, meaning what you do at the top of your head will be reflected into your neo-vagina. Light pressure for two minutes will stimulate and encourage healing of our surgical site. Too much pressure, and you can give yourself a headache. This point's name is derived from the nearly hundred points that meet at that location. I would also encourage light massage on a daily basis, since this point directly influences your new vagina.

Ren 17: *Chest Center*, Ren Mai 17: This is the *Sea of Qi* acupoint, located in the middle of your sternum (Image 21).

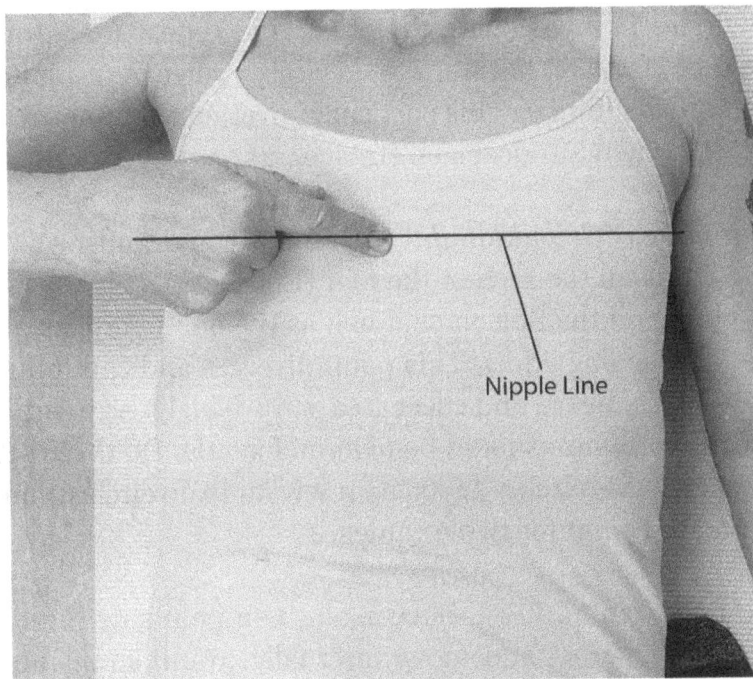

Nipple Line

(Image 21)

This acupoint is inline with the fourth rib on the midline of the body, or the nipple line. Light pressure applied for two minutes or less will benefit how our body gathers Qi, and it benefits your vagina.

Feet and Lower Leg Acupressure

Inner ankle acupoint is where you might need some help those first few weeks, due to your limited range of motion. These acupoints directly influence your new vagina. The pressure should be light and equal to or less than the weight of an orange. The very light pressure is to prevent potential post-op blood clots.

Great Bell, KD-4: This acupoint is located on the inner ankle. As mentioned above, the pressure should be light and gentle. Do nine circles in a clockwise direction, and repeat for a total of three sets. If you do not want to do circles, you can just hold the point for two minutes. This particular divergent channel directly impacts the new surgical site. (Image 22)

Grandmother, Granddaughter (Grandfather Grandson), SP-4: This point is on the arch of the foot (Image 22). It is the fourth of 21 points on the Spleen channel; as the name implies, it has some far reaching effect. This point diverges and can influence your stomach, heart, and chest area, surprisingly. As mentioned above, the pressure should be light and gentle. Do three sets of 9 slow clockwise circles. If you do not want to do circles, you can just hold the point for two minutes.

Woodworm canal, LR-5: once again, Lou points diverge from their main channel and move internally to influence internal aspects that the channel impacts. This point is named after a hole in the bone where blood vessels move in and out to nourish the internal aspect of the bone. Nearly all acupressure points are measured with the width of your own thumb, so this point is located five thumb widths up from your inner ankle bone or (medial malleolus). You can trace this point up the inner or medial shin bone (tibia) until you find a small divot or hole (Image 22).

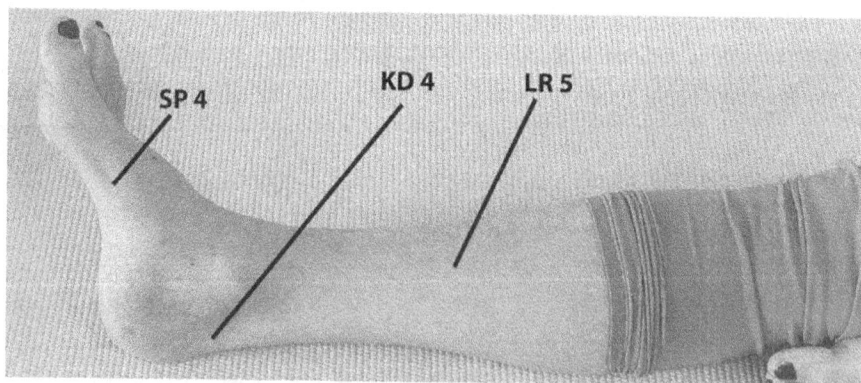

(Image 22)

Foods That Heal

Please be aware that with the full-depth procedures, having soft, loose stools for the first month is important in not aggravating the graft, internal surgical sites and the pelvic floor. Not having large bowel movements or excessive bearing down or pushing during defecation will help prevent fistulas forming between the vaginal cavity and the rectum.

Follow your doctor's complete recommendations when it comes to your digestive tract. With that being said, knowing what foods have healing properties can help in your recovery and healing. We know from the "Helping Yourself Through Recovery " section that pineapple has natural anti-inflammatory properties. Here is a list of some substances that can also help you in your healing process.

- Pineapple - Has natural anti inflammatory properties

- Cut out refined sugars -They will cause inflammation.

- Sweet potatoes nourish the lung tissue.

- Brown rice will nourish the intestinal tract.

- Roasted bone marrow paste - add to soups, it helps build blood.

- Mung beans, found often in Asian grocery stores, will bolster our kidneys.

- Cherry, cranberry, and pomegranate juice helps the urinary tract.

This is a short list along with some other foods and nutritional supplements that can help us heal. Below is a simple and short list I gathered from the Prescriptions for Nutritional Healing book that will help with inflammation.

- Bromelain is pineapple extract and helps with inflammation.

- Three capsules three times a day.

- Eat Fresh Pineapple.

- Drink Aloe Vera juice a few times throughout your week.

- Turmeric teas help reduce inflammation.

- Bone Broth soups help build bone and support a health digestion system.

- Calcium 1200 mg daily (taken with meals and Vit. D3).

- There are two bone support options at Natural Grocers.

- Vitamin A - 25,000 IU daily. (taken with meals)

- Magnesium 1000 MG daily (important in calcium uptake, taken with meals)

- Vitamin C 3,000-6,000 mg daily in divided doses. (taken with meals)

- Vitamin K is essential for bone protein. (taken with meals)

- Zinc: 50 mg daily. (taken with meals)

- Boron: 3 mg. (taken with meals)

- Soy Isoflavones have an estrogenic effect on the body. Estrogen promotes bone mass.

Turmeric: Has also shown that turmeric can decrease inflammation too. Having turmeric tea will help you heal during these first six weeks. There are also Arnica and Turmeric tea found in some natural grocery stores.

Bone Broth: In Chinese medicine, roasted bone broth soups are a wonderful way to help prepare the body for this procedure. As your date comes closer, you may want to incorporate bone broths into your meal structures. You can easily incorporate bone broth into soups. There is also roasted bone broth paste you can purchase that is particularly good in sauces.

Smoothies: There are many of us that may utilize the benefit of smoothies to help us during this time. If it is store-bought, double check the sugar content on the container. If you are into making your own smoothie, adding a little fresh ginger root to your smoothies will help the raw food process better in your gut. Ginger has a natural heating quality and will aid in digestion. This means your body will start to digest and break down nutrients from cold foods more easily while not overtaxing your digestive system.

Nourishing Nuggets

RICE: The Sound Advice.

REST: Ice, Compress, Elevation: These four words are the acronym for the response to sprains, strains, and wounds. It will be useful for us. Ask yourself, what will REST look like? Spend more time horizontal then vertical during the first three weeks.

You will find blood pooling into your pelvic bowl for a few months after this procedure, particularly in the very beginning of your healing. This can in turn cause some pain or discomfort in your surgical site, trouble with dilation, and fluid build up. Do not take a brief trip to the store those first three weeks, even if you are using a cart. Too much vertical pressure can lead to issues later on. Short walks followed by some time spent horizontal is the way to start.

ICE: the surgical site for no more than 20 minutes. Use a reusable ice pack, a bag of frozen peas, or ice cubes in a Ziplock bag. However, always make sure there is a layer between your skin and the ice, as we don't want to cause any tissue damage through direct skin contact with the ice. A pair of shorts or thin towel will do fine.

COMPRESSION: This is a little tricky, but you may find some compression underwear. For me, I picked up some Jockey for Her briefs that I would not mind discarding once the healing has finished. However, they do not provide a lot of compression. One patient told me to buy running shorts that have the inner panty liner, but these also may not provide enough compression. Biking shorts, Spanx, or tight leggings might work better. You can also combine icing with compression shorts for 20 minutes.

ELEVATE: Try to elevate your pelvis above your heart for five to 10 minutes at least once a day, more if you have the time. This can help to move blood back out of the pelvic area after standing or sitting for a while. This can be done with pillows, a yoga block, or several rolled up towels. (Image 23)

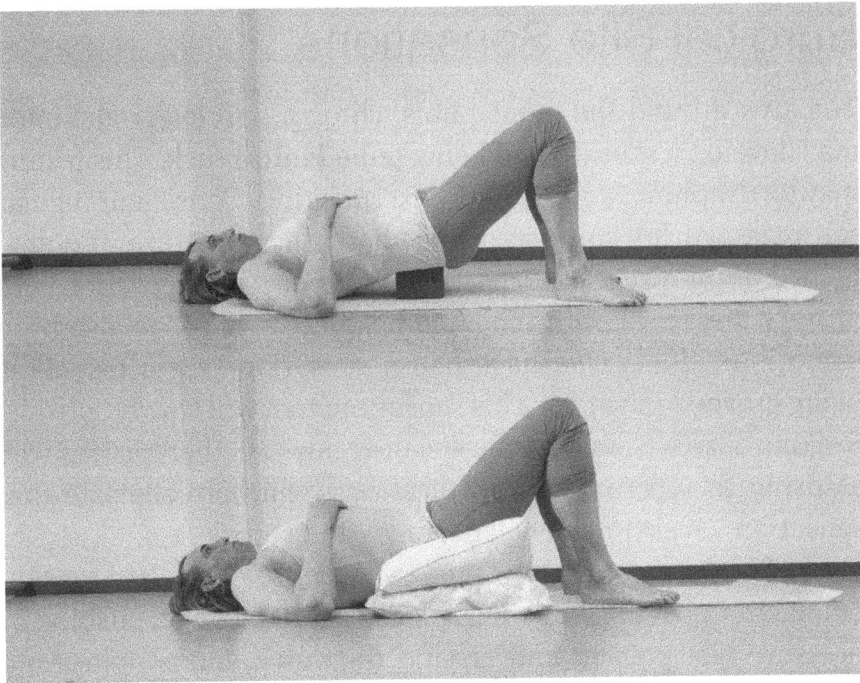

(Image 23)

Your Return Visits

Be prepared for your return visits., be it physical therapy or the surgical nurse and or the surgeon. If you have questions, have them ready. Write them down on your phone or on a notepad. By the second visit to the physical therapist, I had 5 questions on my phone. If you have a problem ANYWHERE or with anything, let them know. You can also send them an email before your visit with your questions.

Due to some gatekeeping some of us have experienced, you may not want to tell them anything. I totally get that reasoning. However, having your key questions ready will help the staff help you. They often have simple fixes that will make your life much easier. Also, you want the best results possible, so ask as many questions as you need in order to get that.

Surgical Site Sensations

The area around the mons pubis, clitoris, and lower abdomen may develop a sensation of being pulled into a tuck. This feeling may be dysphoric and mentally excruciating. Consistent regular self-massage, hot compresses, sitz baths, acupuncture, and time helped minimize this sensation for me. This sensation will **slowly** disappear with time and healing. There have also been some individuals who have had a sensation that a testicle is being crushed or sat on. This sensation, too, will slowly subside. Seeking advice from your physician or physical therapist, as well as using the correct pain medications, will help alleviate that sensation. Over time, it will decrease and stop.

Often, an indicator that your bladder is full will be a pushing or pressure like pain in and around the vulva, mons pubis, and clitoris. You will experience a wide range of new sensations from the surgical site for the first six to eight weeks. Breathe through it, and learn to pay attention to your body. If the pain persists, seek medical attention.

Stenosis

This is a serious issue. It is the narrowing or closing of a specific space, for instance in your case the urethra. The urethra is the tube that runs from your bladder to the outside world and carries urine. The narrowing of the urethra will put you at risk of a urinary tract infection, also known as a UTI. A UTI can bring on the feelings of burning, stinging, pain upon urination or have pink to red tinged urine, seek medical care. There is evidence that pure unsweetened cherry and or pomegranate juice will benefit the urinary tract. Both are very tart and have low sugars. Both will help the kidneys and benefit the bladder, too. It is best to consult your physician, not the interweb.

Isolation

Many of us struggle just to be able to have this procedure. Those of you who may be isolated might not have recognized the larger picture. Having a safe place to return to; Check. Having someone to look in on you while you are healing those first two weeks is IMPORTANT. But many of us may not have someone to take care of us.

Sadly, this isolation is agonizing to so many of us. We may feel like we are totally alone and going through this whole ordeal by ourselves. Finding your pillars of strength around you is vital to your mental health. Seek out those folx prior to surgery to give you strength when you need it most. Build a support system of people so you don't rely on just one person.

If you have access to a support group, you might be able to find people there who want to help you out. Talk to your therapist for more advice on building a team of people. If you want to give yourself some more help, you can contact the Trans Lifeline at 877-565-5800 USA and 877-330-6366 in Canada. For suicide prevention, you may also dial 988 in the USA and Canada.

Immune System

Your immune system will be slightly weakened after this procedure. There are a few things that will help your immune systems recover and will help you reduce inflammation. Below is a simple and short list I gathered from the Prescriptions for Nutritional Healing. These are a good way to help with a compromised immune system.

- L-Lysine 1500 daily.

- Bromelain: 100-500 mg on an empty stomach.

- Vitamin A 25,000 IU daily (if mixed with carotenoids, only take 10,000 IU daily, taken with meals).

- Carotenoids Complex; As directed on the label.

- Vitamin B: Complex 50 mg. (taken with meals)

- Vitamin C 2,000-6,000 daily (over 3,000 may cause diarrhea).

- Zinc 50-100 mg daily. (taken with meals)

- Coenzyme Q10 90 mg daily. (taken with meals)

- Essential fatty acids: As directed on the label

- Vitamin E: 200 IU daily. (taken with meals)

- Acidophilus: (Kyodophius from Wakunaga) 1 tsp on empty stomach twice daily

- Grape seed extract: As directed on the label

- Garlic: (Kyolic from Wakunaga), two capsules three times daily with meals

- Bioavailable multivitamin: As directed on the label (taken with meals)

Please note that adding these supplements with the anti-inflammatory will be too much for the system. Cross reference and combine with the anti-inflammatory nutritional list earlier in this chapter to find a good balance.

Sacred Basin

The word "pelvis" translates from Latin to basin shape. Sacrum translates to the word sacred or holy. Oftentimes, the sacral bone is the last bone to decompose in the human body, so in ancient times, it was thought of as the most important. It may help to look at our pelvis as a "Sacred Basin." We should treat it with kindness, compassion, and caring during the reorganization of our body's tissue and nerves. No trips out that first week, and limit driving to no more than an hour. Be mindful of how much time you have spent up on your feet, and listen to your sacred basin as you heal.

Shallow Depth

This particular procedure will often take less time than full depth procedures, meaning your surgery time will be shorter. However, you can still have many of the issues listed above. They may just be less. For one, you will not have to dilate through your pelvic floor. You will still be able to dilate but not to the extent of those with full depth procedures. Your recovery time is usually cut in half, and many times, you can return to work by fourth week versus sixth. Everything here is still recommended and applies to all those with shallow depth surgery. You can dilate up to about two-to-three inches in depth, and your dilators are not as varied as those folx with full depth. Those first few weeks, there will be potential prolapse of your vagina. This will look like saggy tissue. If this happens, please contact your surgeon or physical therapist. This issue can be fixed with dilation, and if it persists, a revision may be made after nine months to a year.

Chapter 6

Weeks Four Through Six

My emotional roller coaster lasted throughout those first three weeks and into the next three. It was not grief but a sensation of euphoria laced with dysphoria. Sure, the presence of this invasive surgery was still fresh, but the only agonizing feeling was the sensation of being pulled into a surgical tuck. At times it sent me into loops of dysphoria. Some prescribed meds did help ease some of the physical sensation, but not the emotional. Sometimes it felt like a testicle was being sat on; other times, the tension at the upper most sutures was strenuous. For those who have not had to tuck in the past, more power to you. Some of my pre-surgical dysphoria resided in forcing myself into a daily tuck. This unrelenting sensation was present for days and weeks to come. What surprised me was how the regular use of self-acupuncture and massage eased the sensation— sometimes it got rid of it all together. I spoke to a few girlfriends of mine that confided in me about having similar sensations.

Underlying all of these beautiful new sensations, was a ceaseless buzzing and humming sensation right in the clitoral area. At times this sensation had a life of its own. It felt like a button with a continuous buzzing hummmmmm. Honestly, it took me a bit to figure out that it was my clitoris. I was wearing a pad at the time, but I'm pretty sure I had a few micro-orgasms without trying. I suspected that it was mostly due to highly sensitive nerves being relocated. At the time, I did not feel that comfortable poking around down there with the site still so fresh from surgery. With all the discomfort of the sutures, the one thing that felt good was some light direct applied pressure or a hot compress. Much to my delight by the end of these first 6 weeks my clitoris had made itself known!

Those first three weeks, there are so many new sensations that are happening. Nerves striving to reconnect, the brain and endocrine system are managing changes to the body. The one thing never really mentioned prior to this procedure were those oh so delightful NERVE ZINGERS! Thankfully, as an acupuncturist and former massage therapist, I had treated a number of patients with nerve damage. These three weeks are when I really started to benefit the most from self-massage. The arnica ointment I had used post-op had taken care of bruising in just seven days. It was the massage on my inner thighs when I saw half my surgical pain just seep out of the area. From that point forward I'd massage the moment I felt those wildly unpredictable zingers come on. For those who have experienced the discomfort of electrolysis, you may consider it good training wheels for those zingers.

At this point, you are probably ready for an excursion, if you haven't tried it already. I have known some folx who went out and about too early in their first week of recovery and developed an infection around the surgical site, and another person developed some prolapse tissue. Other issues can also arise. Remember to get your rest, no matter how restless you are. Some of your initial swelling has mildly decreased, and walking is easier. Sitting will be difficult for the next three to four months. You are still recovering. You need rest and consistent physical therapy. Let's get the important stuff out of the way.

What Does an Infection Look Like?

Look out for fever, chills, redness, soreness, and/or swelling in the area of surgery or wound. There may be shortness of breath, cough or change in cough, pain, or a burning sensation when urinating. Unusual vaginal discharge or excessive bleeding, new onset of pain, diarrhea, and/or vomiting. This is why it is still so important to make sure you are maintaining your wound care to keep the area as clean as possible.

The pelvic floor has just begun to move forward in the recovery process. The consistent irritation from your daily dilation routine will take months to fully recede. Keep up with your healing thoughts, and continue your anti-inflammation medications as prescribed. Make use of your opiates as needed but remember they are very addictive so use them sparingly.

The continued use of bromelain tablets or capsules and topical Arnica will increase your healing time. If you did not know, you have become an active participant in your recovery with your daily dilation sessions. In this section, massage around the vaginal opening, mons pubis, and inner thigh will ease some of the muscular discomfort. These next few weeks, you will continue to endure the daily annoyance as stitches poke in ways you may not have imagined, and there is some useful advice on that in this chapter. Some of you may be more mobile than others; pace yourself! Infections can arise when you are too active. After those first three weeks, these next three weeks are when you move up in dilation practice and into a new sensation of discomfort.

Emotions

There is an incredible amount of euphoria trimmed with dysphoria during this time period. At this point, I wanted to pull up some tight jeans, but the amount of swelling down in the pelvic area, particularly around the mons pubis and vulva, were all way too much. The continued sensation of being surgically pulled into a tuck will continue during these next three weeks; for some, this may be dysphorically draining. Visually from week one to week six, the surgical site will not look as you expect it to. My friend coined it her "Frankenvagina." I cannot say I appreciate the term, but it was fitting in that it still looks more like a trauma wound rather than a vagina. When you use your mirror during dilation, take time to look around for potential infections and stitches that are poking you. When I was alone with my thoughts, I found writing them down helped. If you have a friend or therapist who can relate and/or can listen to you, this will be extremely valuable. It does help to have a licensed therapist to speak with during these three weeks. Thankfully, the silver lining is, the euphoric sensation that you are complete within your own body always outweighs the dysphoria.

Partnerly advice: If your partner or helper is squeamish about wounds and or blood, you may ask them not to look at your vagina for these first five to six weeks.

Scar Tissue and Healing

For this procedure to be done correctly, there will be quite a few stitches and sutures. Some of us may think that sutures and stitches are the same thing. They are not! Sutures are the threads and or strands used to close a wound. Stitches and/or stitching will refer to the process of closing the wound. Absorbent stitches will slowly dissolve as your wound heals and will not need to be removed. Non-absorbent suture means that sutures will need to be removed at a later date. In this procedure, it is not common for non-absorbent sutures to be used, but check with your surgeon to see if this will be the case with your procedure. In general, there will be three types of thread used for a full depth procedure: thicker thread to secure the internal structures, medium thread for intermediate closures, and the smaller thread used on regions like the labia lips.

With sutures, there will be some form of scar tissue. It is an inevitable part of this process. There will be scar tissue in your grafts, in and around your vaginal opening, your labia lips, your clitoris, and along your groin. Some of this will be internal, and some will be external. Therefore, a majority of postoperative healing lies within the patient's lap—literally and figuratively. In large part, how we heal is up to us. What we eat and don't eat (limiting refined sugars, and alcohol), how we rest, and how we limit toxins such as vaping or smoking tobacco will make a difference. Too much sugar, smoking, processed foods, and too many unsafe healing environments can delay your recovery time. Smoking cigarettes and vaping tobacco products can have a deleterious effect on healing, causing increased scar tissue, limiting blood flow in and out of the wound site, and creating a higher instance of complications to wound healing. Drinking alcohol to excess can also delay healing in your new vagina. Having a conversation with your surgeon about this before surgery and during the first month about these risks is invaluable.

The sutures involved in this procedure will be problematic at times. I have said it earlier and I will say it again—they will poke! They will pull! They will irritate the hell out of you. There are some particularly powerful sutures around the top of your vagina and underneath the Mons pubis. Some will feel the pulling of those stitches for up to six to eight months. The annoying poking and pulling around and in your vaginal opening by sutures is very irritating those first six weeks, but it will vary for everyone. Aloe Vera and your daily padsicles will help soothe those sutures. Something to know is that the internal graft is actually not held in without sutures. This decreases the amount of scar tissue within your vagina. It is your daily dilation that actually keeps the internal aspect of your vagina open. This daily routine assists in adhering your vagina to the internal aspect of the pelvis, as well as creating a cavity capable of penetrative sex.

On more than one occasion, I had a very sharp and painful grabbing sensation near the outer two scars near the inguinal ligament area (Image 24). In my particular case, I woke up 12 hours post-op to excruciating agonizing pain in this region. For me, it felt like I had ripped some internal tissue or suture. You may also experience similar feelings, either immediately after surgery or somewhere along your healing journey. I would encourage a very gentle massage with light pressure in the area, as this will often resolve the discomfort, followed by a hot compress. Another important point is about the extremely powerful suture at the top of your clitoris and around the mons pubis. These first six weeks, when your bladder becomes fuller, you may have a very uncomfortable pushing and or pulling at and around the mons pubis. This pulling and tugging just above your clitoris can be severe at times. There are two things you can do to help you get through these painful and inconvenient times, and they will be discussed next.

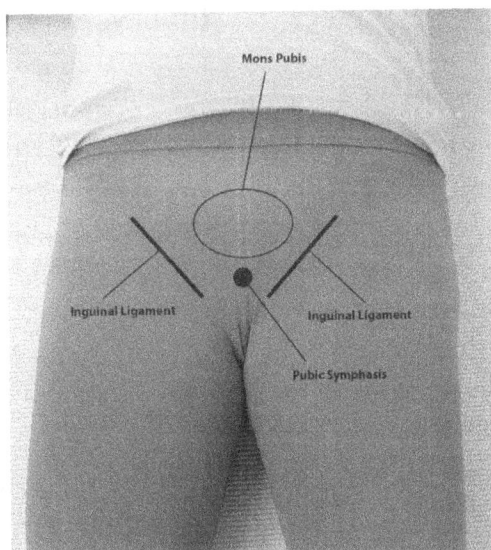

(Image 24)

Caught Stitch, Nerve Zingers, and More

This segment could have easily been in the first 21 day segment, but you had a bunch on your plate those first three weeks. A helpful habit I developed while dilating was to look for any red, puffy, or swollen areas, or wound seepage. It may still not look pretty down there. Reviewing and being on top of what an infection looks like is vital to your health. Keep an eye for any excessive bleeding. Some of you may have wound leakage. When I was performing self-massage, I found a number of areas that were sore under the skin. The physical therapist recommended gentle and light bodywork/massage on those areas. One day during massage I could hear little squishy sounds coming from the right aspect of the vulva due to a pocket of fluid within the wound area. With some self massage and hot compresses the sore spot under the skin decreased and within a few days the squishy sounds stopped completely.

Due to the amount of sensitive surface nerves that were moved around during your surgery you still have nerves finding their way down the healing path. The best way to guarantee long-term healing and recovery of those nerves is with massage. There is a multi-pronged approach to this self-massage. The first is that it increases blood flow to the nerves and surrounding tissue, which will in turn help your immune system. The second prong to the massage approach is to move out all postoperative trauma in the surrounding tissues. When you massage the inner thighs and abdomen these first few weeks, it will move the trauma out of the area allowing other feelings to enter the area. In a few months, this will help you with those first few orgasms, but only after you have moved the surgical trauma out to let the deeper healing begin.

Your nerve zingers and the reawakening of those nerves will go on for the next 12 to 18 months and sometimes longer. Although these sensations are uncomfortable, their presence is a beautiful sign. With every nerve zinger, that means more superficial skin sensations are coming back. Just to warn you, they will go into your clitoris, too. If these sensations are persistent and continued to the point where they interfere with your daily functioning, you need to consult your physician to ease the symptoms. There have been a few patients who have come into my office with a sensation of a crushed former testis. The sensation is quite unpleasant and dysphoric. Consult your physician, as there are some medications that may be helpful with these sensations. Aggravated nerves respond well to moist heat, so you may try applying a hot compress to the area to ease the sensations.

Sitz Bath and Padsicles

If you have not yet utilized the Sitz bath, please do so. This is the primary way to keep your wound site clean and disinfected. Besides, it is your vagina's personal hot tube. Even though the surgical wound is in the process of healing, it is not healed yet—so practice your Sitz baths. In time your daily Sitz bath will minimize your scar too. Your well-intentioned kindness, care, and compassion is key at this point to your healing and recovery, so think good thoughts about your vagina when you are taking that sitz bath. During this time period, you will transition to a smaller pad and move away from the bulky overnight pads. This will be your time to become an expert on all things about menstrual pads. Find what works, regarding length, thickness, wings, etc. I will suggest choosing "long" or "extra long" pads, as there will still be seepage from multiple wounds ranging from your clitoris to your vaginal opening. Once you make that switch to smaller pads, you will notice an improved difference in your comfort. If you experience irritation because of the pad size, that will decrease, and smaller pads are just more comfortable to wear.

However, just because you have downsized to a smaller or thinner pad does not mean you need to discontinue your Padsicles or other skin and wound care. The skin around the wound and neo-vagina still needs your care and attention. It will still be itchy, and there will always be a stitch poking around. Keep up with the aloe vera and bacitracin to moisturize the drying skin and soothe healing.

Expect your discharge to continue—as long as you are dilating and douching, you will have some discharge. There is external tissue that has been brought into a new environment; part of this adaptation will be the slothing of the epidermis. Douching does reduce discharge but does not completely eliminate it. You will still have some pink blood on your pad either from dilation or an angry suture. Continued application of a padsicle cocktail of aloe vera and bacitracin will keep the tissue moist and pliable. Between week six or eight, you will probably discontinue using padsicles. But you are in control; if you want to use them longer, you do you. It will help to discontinue the use of bacitracin after eight weeks since the risk of infections has decreased, but feel free to continue to use Aloe Vera. At this point, you have become familiar with douching; keep up the practice. This will become a weekly component for the coming years.

Dilation Talking Points

There are some talking points around dilation that can be discussed now. Dilation is how you will keep your vagina from closing and/or shortening—as that is what the body will naturally want to do to your beautiful new anatomy. In these next few weeks, you may move up in dilators size. Unfortunately, it will hurt—at least it did for me! Finding what works for you is your key to success. If you are not interested in penetrative sex, you do not have to go up in size if you do not want to. That being said, your body will still want to close up any new holes, so it is important to keep dilating with at least the smallest size. Stay studious with your three times a day routine and do your best to not skip any sessions.

Around now you may want to investigate the variety of dilators out on the market. It is IMPORTANT to make sure they are designed specifically for vaginoplasty recovery. There are ones that are hard plastic and ones that are more pliable. Explore your options as you will be dilating for years to come. It is also important to note that no matter what dilator you are using, it is imperative to wash it after each use. This will prevent infections—and you do not want an infection in your new vagina! If you are using hard plastic dilators, it is not a bad idea to put them through the dishwasher every month or so to completely disinfect them. If you are using other dilators, please read the recommendations on how to thoroughly clean them.

As you begin this healing stage, there are some things on the horizon that you may need to consider in regards to dilation. Not all people want penetrative sex; some do and others do not. This is completely up to you, and you should never feel pressured into something you do not wish to do. Nor should peer pressure make you feel that you are any less authentic. But, know if you have not prepared with a larger dilator, penetrative sex will be painful when you attempt it in the future. As a side note, you probably will not be cleared to have sex until three months after surgery, but check with your own surgeon regarding when this is OK.

At this point in your dilation practice, the repetitiveness is painful, monotonous, and time-consuming. Finding the correct position while working through the unpleasantness is not easy.

I think it is important to discuss the number of benefits to a consistent dilation schedule because at this point, you might begin to question just how committed to this you are. Firstly, it helps educate the pelvic floor muscle group. This muscle group is experiencing something—so new that it will take time for it to fully adjust. Dilating teaches the brain to experience a completely new sensation. The action of dilation stimulates the brain and body to send blood to the area to help with the recovery process. The natural healing process is telling the pelvic floor muscle group to close up that hole,so regular dilation prevents the natural act of closure by the body.

Over time this routine dilation of the pelvic floor will prevent closure. It is important to listen to your body during this healing process. Pain is a language your body uses to inform the brain there has been trauma. This begins the healing process, but like a skilled dancer, we want to train the body and muscles to do something new. It takes time, patience, and focus. When dilating into wider and deeper depth, you may experience pulling on the vulva and clitoris; this is just one aspect of listening to your body. Using lidocaine and your pain medication will help some of this.

Why is it uncomfortable? The graft used to create the internal aspect of your vagina is scrotal tissue and penile tissue, both of which are inherently very sensitive. This increased sensitivity, surrounded by aggravated pelvic floor muscle groups and the natural inflammation process of a healing body will generally cause pain. While there was a lot of hands-on learning those first 21 days, now is the time to find what works best for you, not just physically but mentally as well. If you are assiduous with your physical therapy/dilation it will pay off after 15 weeks. Finding the time now will make it easier later in your recovery process.

One other facet to consider to our discomfort is what we eat. This may be anecdotal, but it should be considered. The deeper you dilate, the closer we are to some of our small intestines. Your intestine and gut organs have the same inflammation qualities as the exterior of our bodies. If you have food allergies, it will cause the small intestine to become inflamed. If you are eating excess refined sugars, gluten, or dairy, some of these foods will also cause gut inflammation. Being aware of your food intake is important these first six weeks. I am sensitive to dairy products, and I found that when I had too much of it, the dilation pain was worse. When I cut back on the amount of cheese I was eating, the dilation was easier. So if there are foods that make you feel bloated or cause you some gastrointestinal discomfort, try cutting back on them during the early stages of healing.

You may dilate for the recommended time or for longer if you can tolerate it. Sometimes I would stretch out my pelvic floor between dilators and give my pelvic floor a breather. Something to expect when you move up in dilators is that you will have some pink blood and increased pain during wider dilation sessions. Using lidocaine will make a world of difference. Remember to keep buying your recommended lube in advance, you will need it. Refer back to Pre-dilation stretches in Chapter 1.

One sensation you might develop that does go away with regular physical therapy is the stretching and rope burning pain that happens with wider dilators. This is your time to engage in breathing techniques and to learn to pull out the dilator when it becomes too much and add more lube. Give your pelvic floor a little stretch if it becomes too painful. Have patience and stick with it, even if it takes a little longer. This burning or stretching pain can go on for at least six to10 weeks when increasing dilator width. Use your lidocaine prior to your dilation session.

Personally I want to say around five and a half to six months, the dilation pain diminished significantly. Between the seventh and eighth month, it was gone altogether, thankfully (YIPPPEEEEE). Those first 4 months, talk to your doctor about using some lidocaine gel to assist with the pain and make dilation a more tolerable activity, particularly if you are getting to the point of wanting to skip sessions due to the discomfort.

This is not the time to pull up your big girl pants and work through the pain. This stretching or widening can be excruciating—breathe and do not force something if you are not ready. Go at your own pace, and do what works for you. Surprisingly, due to the discomfort of the dilation and the variety of sutures, some of my patients were having subtle orgasms from the pulling and tugging of their clitrois. Some may develop some pre-cum in and around your ureter. For me, this was incredibly affirming and validating, as cisgender women also get wet during stimulation. This is a nice bonus for suffering through dilation, but it may not happen for everyone.

Since we are reeducating the pelvic floor, some of us will experience some internal pelvic floor pain. This will feel like pain on the inside or your vaginal cavity, it could be at any area of the circumference of your vagina, felt deeply or near the opening. I cannot emphasize how having access to a pelvic floor physical therapist is important. If there is one thing that we all need in those post-op days, weeks, and months, is an increase in pelvic floor physical therapy. The light at the end of the tunnel is that it does become easier after five months. If access to a physical therapist is not possible, you can help ease your pelvic floor discomfort by utilizing pre-dilation stretching prior to your dilation sessions. You may also find using the smallest dilator inserted halfway and doing GENTLE small circles around the inside of your vagina to massage some of those pelvic floor muscles. This has helped some of my patients with ongoing pelvic floor discomfort.

It is OK to get tired of dilating. Around 15 weeks post-op, I came down with COVID-19, an omicron variant. One night, I became so exhausted from the process of dilation that I only did it for nine minutes and cried nearly the whole time. My physical therapist was amazingly sympathetic and said, "It is OK to be tired of it." At some point, you will probably find yourself feeling fed up with the whole process. During these difficult times, lidocaine and distraction can be extremely useful. It does get easier, so hang in there and do the best you can. Finding what works best for you at this stage will make a huge difference to the future of your dilation practice.

Post-Surgical Sensations

Now, many of you may have felt something else buzzing during your last three weeks. There may be a buzzing, humming feeling in your clitoris. One of the most beautiful aspects of this procedure is your clitoris. At times, it will feel like an oversized button pushing and humming away as it heals. Sometimes, the buzzing is there, and other times it is not. During all of your healing and recovery you will want to **apply light** and very gentle pressure to the region of your clitoris and vulva. Too much pressure and your body will push back with pain. Become comfortable touching yourself gently down there, through your clothing or with a towel, with gloves or with clean hands. That touch will go a long way four months down the road. At times it may feel like a large button other times it will be a light hum. Over time it will decrease in size but not necessarily sensation. Begin to explore it ever so gently, not trying to find sexual arousal, but to learn what sensation it has and how sensitive it is.

This is the same region that contributes to the regular tugging or pulling sensation that may feel similar to being "tucked." This persistent sensitivity at times can cause some dysphoric feelings and can be overwhelming. You may find laying down and getting the blood away from the pelvic floor eases some of that sensation. Remember, this is just part of the healing process. It will not feel like this forever. Try to breathe through it.

Let's touch on this possibility of dysphoria. For some, there may be a continued surgical discomfort and swelling around the mons pubis, vulva, clitoris, and pubic symphysis. This swelling and recent surgery sensations may cause dysphoria. This tugging feeling along your underwear lines is miserable for some. It will help to have someone to talk to about it professionally. It has been asked of me numerous times: When will the tension, pulling, and tugging sensation end? The area of the mons pubis and pubic symphysis is holding a tremåendous amount of surgical tension. Even though you may be experiencing visual euphoria by looking down and seeing the natural "V" pattern, there may still be some continued dysphoria due to the internal healing process still trying to move fluid out of the area and get accustomed to everything being in a new position. This region will remain tight, tender, swollen, and sensitive to the touch. Topically adding Arnica at least two to three times daily is great and will help. If you have pubic hair, lightly massage over it by using high quality, unscented massage oil such as grape seed. Work in the region of the mons pubis and inguinal area. Consider getting or continuing the use of compression shorts during this period.

You now have the body that fits with your heart and soul. Over the next few months, there is a grace and calm that pours throughout your soul. But there is one more facet that needs to be added to the healing table. Your clits will buzz, humm, and ZING. The number of nerves that are regenerating into your pelvis, vulva, and clitoris will cause nerve zingers for a number of months. I have known patients to get nerve zingers well into their second year of healing. The zingers will be in the labia lips, the clitoris itself, the vulva, and the mons pubis. These zingers will double you over. They are painful, but it is more of the surprise way in which they come on. You may drop to one knee with surprise pain or pinching. Most times, the discomfort leaves as fast as it arrived. This is just another aspect of the body healing. Surprisingly, only a few individuals reported these nerve zingers into the full depth of the graft region. **Consider yourself warned.**

During this three week period of healing, you will be desperately wanting and able to get out and about. This increased moving and standing will result in more blood flow into your pelvic floor. This will consequently result in some discomfort and perhaps swelling. This is a prime reason NOT to go back to work or perform long standing or lifting chores. Your minimum lifting capacity is no more than 10 pounds those first six weeks. Even for folx with a shallow depth procedure, your turnaround time is four to six weeks. In this time frame, your use of the donut will increase. Be mindful of how much you use it, because this will cause increased pressure and a pooling of blood in your new genitals. If used for too long, or to excess, you may develop hard, tough, leathery skin all around the surgical site. Finding the time and space to ELEVATE your pelvis by putting a pillow under your butt or at least lay down (preferably fully horizontal) for a few minutes will be beneficial.

Ice will continue to help with the inflammation through these 21 days. Please note that some inflammation will persist for the next five months. COMPRESSION is useful when laying down by gently adding one to two pounds of pressure on and around your mons pubis and vulva. Interestingly, you may actually find it uncomfortable due to the swelling in the region to wear a pair of tight jeans or slacks. With either the shallow or full depth procedure, REST should still be on your radar. Listen to your body, it will let you know when you have done too much. You will get tired easier, and you may not feel as rested when you do wake up. These are your cues to get some REST and take it easy.

Hot Compress

In my surgical notes, it suggests using a hot compress to help with the surgical site. The first 21 days, I was very nervous about infection and did not utilize a hot compress. My concerns were warranted, but the first time I applied that hot compress, I melted_t felt so good. Generally, people may start to use a hotpack after the first seven days. As your wound site heals, there are times when a hot compress will be favored over an ice pack. The hot compress will soothe various suture lines and tension. At this point, it may help move some fluid out of the area especially as you continue to practice massage. If you add it prior to your dilation times, this may ease these first few moments of discomfort during expansive aspects of dilation.

There are individuals who used a hot compress sooner. Using a hot compress along with your daily sitz bath will increase your healing and recovery. To create a hot compress, rinse a washcloth in hot water (ensure it is not too hot) and place it between your legs with some sort of barrier between it and your skin. A kitchen towel or even just your underwear will work. You do not want to scald the area, so be very careful. A method that I used was to wrap a wet, very hot, washcloth inside a dry towel and then put it on my genitals. I could still enjoy the warmth but didn't have to worry about scalding myself. Refer to image 13 in Chapter 3.

Massage and Breaking Down Physical Dysphoria

These next three weeks, you will want to focus on what would be considered Swedish massage techniques. For someone who has 16,000 hours of massage experience, I can assure you that there are great benefits that come from self-massage. The more familiar you are with touching around your new vagina is important. This touch can help slowly break down the dysphoric barrier we had placed around our formal genitalia and the region it had resided in. This compassionate touching and massaging will break down muscle memory trauma. The added bonus I have not told you is a gift that comes after the three-month mark. From this simple, gentle, and compassionate caring touch will be some really great orgasms later on down the road. For me, this part of transitioning was surprisingly powerful psychologically. Once the shades are pulled back, some new, beautiful sensation comes forward. This will be different for everyone, particularly after seeing your vagina slowly transform from a swollen, injured surgical site into your new vagina. Believe in yourself; your body will follow.

Touch is an incredible component to these next few weeks of healing, including sexual healing. Some of us may feel instantly fulfilled; for others it may be a long time coming. Healing comes at your own pace. Becoming comfortable and familiar with regular massaging of the legs and abdomen the first three weeks onward will allow you to be more at home with touching yourself more intimately these next few weeks and months.

For this particular three-week period, it will be to your advantage to stay with the previous chapter's massage therapy information. If you have only done self-massage once a week in those first 21 days, that small amount of care will increase blood flow to the wound site and help remove post-surgical lymphatic fluid. Massage has shown to speed up healing and decrease your recovery time. Keeping up with some massage therapy the first six weeks will help you immensely when you start back to work.

Every massage stroke or some gently applied pressure to an area that feels swollen or hurt will help with how your body feels its new self. By applying light pressure, you immediately activate a surface nerve response. This sets off a whole set of sensory mechanisms within your brain. Knowing you can help yourself with just a small understanding of the benefits of self-care will help in your current circumstances. If you have applied just a few self-massage days, you may have inevitably found the numb patch or patches of surface tissue as mentioned earlier. Applying some arnica and some light massage to that region regularly along with a hot compress will bring back that sensation. Have patience, as these nerves take a while to heal.

Professionally, I have treated patients with nearly no surface nerves sensations for months. Then, on a follow up appointment, I will perform a surface nerve test, and to my surprise, half of the area that was damaged is nearly back to normal. Nerves take time to heal, and a compassionate touch to lull them awake.

IMPORTANT
To maintain a healthy surgical site, latex, nitrile, or vinyl **gloves are REQUIRED the first eight weeks.** This is to keep the surgical site clean and prevent infection.

There are concerns when performing strokes that are too deep during your massage. The biggest concern is a blood clot. Blood clots come from blood that has turned into solid form rather than remaining liquid. This hardened blood is then worked loose inside a vein or an artery can move into the heart and or the brain. With all of the localized inflammation in your body, the risk is there. Let the surface skin be your internal guide to pressure used during your massage time. Anything greater than one pound comes with a risk.

Shallow Depth and Back to Work

The vast majority of this book is around full depth procedures. There are those who will receive a shallow depth surgery. With this particular surgery, patients are often allowed to go back to work by the fourth week. This is not an easy feat. I would encourage you to read the rest of the next chapter on back-to-work planning. Even though you may have had a shallow depth procedure, this is no reason to believe you are finished. There are a number of issues that will still accompany you into your next 10 months of recovery. Those with a shallow depth procedure you will still find the next few chapters to be a great benefit.

Return Visits

During these three weeks, you will get to experience the miserable sensation of the infamous SPECULUM. This is a medical device that is inserted into your vagina and then expanded. It allows the medical practitioner to examine the internal aspect of your vagina. Prior to this procedure, I had heard stories from patients and friends. Now, if you have been dilating as you should be, having an object inserted into your new vag is nothing new by this point. However, it will be that moment the practitioner expands the speculum that will have your eyes pop wide with a new experience. It is important for the medical staff to see that the inside of your vagina is healing well and look for any potential fistulas or internal issues. For some, it is painful, for others it isn't, but whatever the case is for you, it will certainly be a sensation you have not encountered before.

Pad Irritation Advice

There may come a time when you are in between pads, pantyliners, and no pads. If you don't wear a pad after dilation, your underwear becomes rather wet or damp. This is not that unpleasant, but it does have the potential to lead to a rash or jock itch. Upon telling this issue to my surgeon at one of my follow-up appointments, they suggested placing a swatch of cloth (rather than a pad) in my underwear to absorb any potential liquid. They suggested a t-shirt material or other soft fabric. Sometimes the extended use of pads can irritate the skin. I cut up an old, clean t-shirt making about 10 swatches to try out. They worked surprisingly well— an hour, pull it out and discard it. The cotton was much easier on the skin.

Dietary Inflammation

Dietary inflammation many times is something we can not see, and far worse, you do not always feel. The vagus nerve that innervates the gut does not have the tactile sensations surface nerves are instilled with. Intestinal tract inflammation is very common particularly when eating refined sugars, highly processed foods, or having food sensitivities such as soy, lactose or gluten intolerance. The irritation that happens inside the intestinal tract may go on for days at a time. For some of my patients including myself, inflammatory foods may lead to some deeper tenderness during dilation.

Granulation

Yes, that dirty word is back in your life. During these three weeks you will still have the potential to develop granulations. This issue afflicts a number of individuals during these first six weeks. The first time it happened, I walked straight to the scheduler and made another appointment. It was a proactive measure on my behalf. Granulation is removed with silver nitrate; at first I thought it would hurt to have it removed. Much to my surprise, when the nurse practitioner applied it to the granulation, it felt better. This is a healthy response to your healing; take it as a good omen–It means you are healing. With each follow-up, the granulations will diminish, and you will never notice it again. Now, if they could only do that with the dilation pain.

Movement and Range of Motion

There is something that caught me by surprise, and that was the limited range of motion I had in my pelvic region, specifically when bending at the waist. Simply bending over to pick something up or tying your shoes will be limited. Let pain and the body's limited range of motion be your STOPPING signal. PLEASE do not try to push past those limitations. The risk of tearing and hurting some internal suture can lead to pain and a delay in recovery. The lack of mobility in your waist and pelvis will decrease and you will see noticeable changes with improved movability between nine to 12 months. It may help to refer back to Chapter 1 stretches to assist you in your recovery.

Chapter 7

Weeks Seven through Nine

One morning I woke up and looked back in order to take stock of where I was. I had reached the top of the mountain for any major complications. I felt positive for what lay ahead. Firstly, I survived a very invasive surgery. Secondly, I passed the pee test, and lastly, no infections. It felt like I had been through a gauntlet in an adventure story. All my electrolysis was good training practice for learning how to deal with the persistent pain of dilating. My brother and I used to give each other rope burns on the forearm as little kids, a version of "who could take the most pain!" I found this dilating pain was very similar. I am not sure if I should thank my brother or not.

Work was on my mind; I had made a few test runs to work and back. I had even spent a few hours at the office to simulate the upcoming work environment. It seemed OK; the commute home was always uncomfortable, though. By the end of a few hours, my pelvic floor was raw with pain, swelling, and, worst of all, with increased nerve zingers, ugh. Having one of those in traffic is a no joke. Much to my dislike, I continued with tylenol or ibuprofen to lessen the painful drive home. I was always glad to see that large gloriously cold ice pack when I arrived and/or a nice hot compress, whatever my vagina ordered for the day.

Dilating at the end of your work day SUCKS! I knew individuals who just kept utilizing the smaller dilator and/or they stopped their second dilation session all together. In my years leading up to my surgery, I had spoken to physical therapists who had to work on individuals who stopped dilating in the U.S. and Europe. The rehabilitation was excruciating or a revision was required, with a return to the three times a day dilation schedule. I did not have time for that in my life, so I made myself keep dilating.

After a few "dress rehearsals" to work, I turned back to my trusty pre-flight checklist and started over, this time focusing on my concerns for work. Once I had identified my personal needs and concerns, I knew I had a good game plan for the next three weeks. I did have the tremendous fortune of going back part-time without all the demands of full-time work. However, at the end of every day there was always the misery of dilation. I was a skilled bodyworker with a keen understanding of what trauma and surgery can do to an individual, yet what I was experiencing was unclear to me. There was this continued presence of pulled skin and tissue right at my mons pubis and vulva; at times it was unbearable. Surprisingly, it always felt better after a hot compress. This is when I realized they must have used a very powerful suture to secure the top of my vulva and clitoris. I mentioned it to the physical therapist once. They had not heard anyone else mention it before me, which was a little frustrating, as it left me to figure it out on my own.

Despite being back up on my feet and at work, I could sense these next few weeks would be a struggle. I did self-massage as often as possible during my work week. As much as I wanted to go out on weekends, to be in nature or shoot a round of billiards, my pelvis needed to heal and rest. Many times on weekends I'd limit my time out and often came home early to lay down and rest. Being conscious of discomfort and swelling during this time is important. Too much time up on your feet has the potential to send you home for a few days of bedrest, and most of us cannot afford to take any more time off.

It will help to use the pre-flight list, along with the things in this chapter, to assist you as you head back to work. You are still recovering; please remember that. I have mixed feelings personally and professionally regarding the length of time suggested for the recovery. Out of respect for how much our pelvic floor does (especially for the full-depth surgery), this recovery time could easily be eight weeks. Many of us just do not have the time or the money saved up to take 60 days off.

During these next three weeks, getting around may feel nice, but it may come with some pushback from your healing vagina. Problems may arise with too much of a workload, too much time on your feet, sitting for too long, or lifting too much. Pacing yourself and listening to your body will be an important part of this healing phase. There are some wonderful benefits from a few sessions of manual lymph drainage by a professional. A light, full-body massage may be a nice gift for yourself. If you have been steadfast with your dilation, this pays off with a decrease in your dilation times.

Back to Work

Back to life, back to reality. This may sound easy and even exciting; after all, you have been cooped up for six weeks. Hopefully you have done some simple walks and have been able to spend more time on your feet and sitting with the use of a cushion. However, please be aware that it is not as easy as it sounds, and it won't be for a few more months. If you have the ability to work part time for the first three weeks back to work, that will help tremendously. Or if you have the ability to work from home, where you can more comfortably position yourself, that will be helpful as well.

These next few weeks back into the swing of things will take time. You will need to listen to what your body is capable of at this point. Pushing through it is not a good approach right now. I repeat: pushing through pain is not healthy. This is often the time individuals reduce or stop dilating twice daily because of the tremendous amount of pain from the inflammation, the day's use, and lack of time. You may try taking icing and taking an NSAID (ibuprofen) an hour before dilating, or taking a prescribed muscle relaxant will help the pelvic floor. Check in with your doctor or physical therapist for some professional advice. I had mentioned above to consider a little pre-flight checklist for these next two months. Let us take inventory, shall we?

- You will still have to dilate at least twice a day, if not three times.

- There is the drive and or commute to work, as well as back home, to consider if you don't work remotely.

- You will need to find a place at work to lay down (preferably) or at least get your feet up for a while.

- Standing vs. sitting: If your office is not equipped with a versatile ergonomic desk that allows for standing and sitting options, you will want to ask for it.

- If you do not work at a desk, are there other accommodations you can make so you are not on your feet for the whole shift?

- Just because you can sit with a neck or donut cushion does not mean you will want to. Excessive use of the cushions may cause some issues to arise such as increased swelling, zingers and tightness.

- Getting in and out of a car, bus, train, or light rail.

- If your commute has any large bumps or you are constantly jostled.

- How much time are you going to be on your feet walking, lifting, moving?

One thing that is important to remember during these next few weeks is to watch how much lifting or carrying you are doing these next 45 days. When you lift and carry something heavy, your pelvic floor is working more than ever. The pelvic floor, along with your abdominal muscles and erector muscles in your back, are there to maintain your posture during the whole lifting and carrying process. If lifting and carrying is done repetitively throughout your work day, this can lead to a great deal of inflammation, which in turn may complicate dilation at the end of your day. The longer you sit down during your commute, be it by car, bus, train, or plane, even with the donut or neck cushion, this will also lead to a swollen vaginal cavity. If your commute involves excessive jostling, the return trip home can be miserable at times.

When it comes to those folx who work at a desk, a more comfortable chair with height options will be best. One patient was able to have an ergonomic workstation installed at their desk upon their return, allowing them to sit or stand while working on their computer. Another installed it at her home work station. There will be times when standing is far easier than the up and down of an office chair. Not to mention, for the next four months, there can be a limited range of motion when you are bending over at the waist.

Professionally, I would suggest when going back to work that you put some thought and care into what you are asking of your body. Be a compassionate healer for your own recovery. The donut cushion will cause blood to pool; this will consequently cause your labia and surgical site too swell. With constant usage these next three weeks, the skin may become very leathery due to swelling and the lack of good fluid movement through your pelvis. I have seen this with my patients and with myself. It is very dysphoric and emotionally scary. You can move the blood and ease the discomfort by just elevating your pelvis. This will cause an increase in blood flow into the area and a relief of the tension. A hot compress will usually ease swelling and discomfort. In fact, you may find yourself alternating a lot between an icepack to help the swelling decrease and a hot compress to help the blood move fluid out of the area.

The reality is that lifting, traveling, moving, standing, sitting, and shifting increases blood flow into your pelvis, and this will make it very painful to dilate. Going back to work will zap your energy, as your stamina is not back to 100 percent. The takeaway from this conversation is that not only will you be going back to work, but you will still need to dilate two or three times a day. Finding some time to elevate your pelvis, ice the region, or add a hot compress will prepare your vagina for your daily physical therapy routine.

Pelvic Sensations, Floor, and Dilation

You will continue to experience a consistent pulling and tugging of tissue and skin around your mons pubis. This will be very persistent for the next few months. In some cases, individuals have felt this sensation well into the fifth and sixth month marks. During your surgery, those upper sutures were sewn in with very powerful sutures. They are there to keep your tissue together, but they can cause significant tugging due to their strength. This will not cause you to have too many walking issues, but it may be hard to bend at the waist for the next three months. Massage on the mons pubis and vulva region can ease this feeling, as well as getting your feet and pelvis elevated.

Despite being up and about, gravity is not your friend at this point. As much as your heart pumps blood throughout the body, it needs some help getting all of the extra swelling and fluid out of the pelvic region. Knowing when to get off of your feet if the pressure becomes too much is important. This sensation of pulling/tugging will often be steady until you get your feet and pelvis up. This issue is not limited to those working on their feet, but also to those sitting for long periods of time. There is still a fair amount of internal inflammation despite the initial three weeks of discomfort having decreased.

With all this increased activity and commuting, you will find the pelvic floor to be very hard to dilate through. At the same time, you are often moving up in dilator sizes. This can be painful for all of that delicate tissue, particularly at the end of your day. I cannot repeat this enough: You will want to have a lidocaine ointment prescription. During these three weeks, you may want to spend about 10 minutes prior to your second dilation session stretching.

Opening up the pelvic floor and elevating it prior to dilation will ease some of the discomfort. Take your time, and breathe during your session. There will be a rope burn sensation when going up in sizes of dilators. When you increase dilators, you will most likely also have some pink blood at the end of your dilation session. I repeat this in each section, but it is important to find your rhythm, find your solace, your happy place. Use your VR device,; turn up the music, or find some other distraction. My partner would often join me in the bedroom and we would chat just like we were in the kitchen together to help keep my mind off of the dilation pain and burning sensations. Find what works for you, and keep at it. You are making great progress with your dilation, and it is hard work but well worth it.

Throughout the following months, you will be encouraged to increase your dilator size. This is not to just help with depth but also with the width of your vagina. When you first get your dilators, you may look at them in excitement, but when you see the largest of the dilators, you may not believe it will be possible. At times, moving up to a larger dilator may appear daunting and might look unachievable, and I will unfortunately tell you, the larger dilators will hurt! Once again, have patience, and breathe throughout the whole process. If you find dilating extremely painful, you may ask to be prescribed muscle relaxants to calm the pelvic floor. If you are using lidocaine, make sure to apply it five to10 minutes ahead of time to let it do its work before you start trying to dilate. Go at your own pace and breathe through it. You may find a sitz bath before dilation to be helpful. The warmth of the water will help the tissues become softer and pliable. The warmth will also help your underlying pelvic floor muscles relax.

Becoming familiar with the pre-dilation pelvic floor openers and adductor stretch will ease some dilation discomfort. You also have hip rotator muscles that come very close to your neo-vagina. Besides myself I have known a few friends and patients that had some small issues with their rotator muscles being aggravated during dilation. This is another great reason to familiarize yourself with some of the previous chapters stretches. There is an additional simple exercise you can do while preparing for dilation. This basic muscle movement is known as the "Windshield Wiper" exercise. Lay yourself down on your bed with legs together and feet pointing up. Now rotate your feet so your toes are pointed to the sides, and then rotate your feet back together (Image 25). You do not need to hold the position, just pretend your feet are windshield wipers. Repeat 10 times.

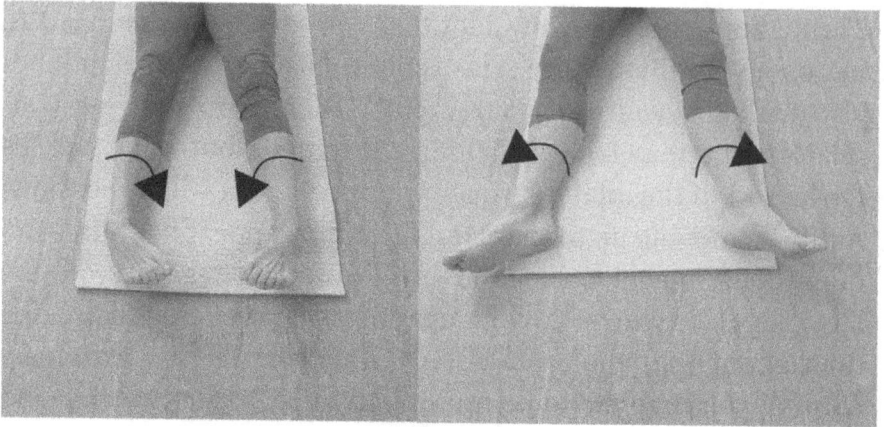

(Image 25)

As you may have noticed, after the first dilation session there will be some residue in your underwear. Having this daily extra moisture down there is not that great for your skin. During those first six weeks establishing a consistent douching habit will start to pay off for you now. You may try douching after your evening dilation to prevent this from getting to be too much during the night. However, don't be surprised you may have to swap out your undies in the middle of the night to stay dry down there. On more than one occasion, I have had patients who developed a form of jock itch or a simple rash due to the increase in moisture. Keeping that area dry will help prevent jock itch or a rash.

Massage Therapy and Self-Care Techniques

To this point, you have learned the important gentle light massage stroke in the previous chapters. If all you wanted to do was just that light massage, you would be absolutely fine. With that being said, I am going to go a little more in depth in this section on ways to help your pelvic floor after a day on your feet. So the more comfortable you are with self-massage, the easier these techniques will be. This type of massage therapy is when you can focus more on the external aspect of the vaginal area and begin to work on the scar tissue associated with the surgery. The mons pubis will still be tender and swollen. Continuing to apply arnica ointment or gel to the area will be beneficial, as will the gentle massage from the previous chapters. The areas of massage to focus on now will be the upper, inner thigh region and closer to your vagina. We will also cover a few more acupoints around the lower abdomen and pubic symphysis. Knowing where the scar tissue is and how to care for this healing tissue is a great aid to your recovery.

Now that you are past the major infection stages, you may begin to address scar tissue massage in greater detail. There is tissue right around your vaginal opening that could use your assistance. As discussed in the previous chapter, those effleurage massage strokes will speed up healing. Now that we are in a safe healing zone around week six, you can do light, gentle circles directly on each scar. The pressure is equal to one pound, so very light and soft in nature. If you have worked all day and you are scheduled to dilate, a sitz bath or a hot compress will soothe the area prior to massaging. Spend just seven to 10 minutes doing gentle slow circles on either side of your vagina. The area will be sore from having been on your feet or sitting upright all day. The tissue around the vagina may be tight or swollen and feel tough. These light, circular massages can be extended onto your upper inner thighs. These massages are meant to be soft enough to bring blood flow into the area, but not deep enough to cause swelling by irritating the tissues that are healing underneath.

The sutures that have made up your labia lips could use some soft, compassionate attention. When I first did this I could not believe how good it felt, and not in a sexual way, but in a tissue relief way. Use a small, hand-held mirror to help you find those exact suture lines if needed. Gently, and with a compassionate touch, lightly glide one finger up it from bottom to top. Using massage oil and arnica mix, I would suggest three times a week in this area during these threeweeks. If you do not have arnica, try using some massage oil or unscented lotion. Let's go over the bodywork below.

Massage Therapy Weeks Six Through12

Position: Just like in Chapter 2, place or position yourself on your back with legs in butterfly position (knees open bottom of feet together) or with feet flat and your knees bent. You may want to lay on a towel, just in case you get some oil on your sheets. Presumably you will be in a bed or on the floor when doing a self massage.

1. As before, have your Arnica ointment or gel ready, along with a little massage oil.

2. Remember to <u>wash and or snitize</u> your hands before and after any type of bodywork.

3. Circular Effleurage around vaginal opening: Rather than long strokes, we will be doing very small circles around your vaginal opening. The pressure can be the weight of two oranges, or two pounds of pressure. Repeat on either side of your vaginal opening three times before moving to the labia. (Image 26)

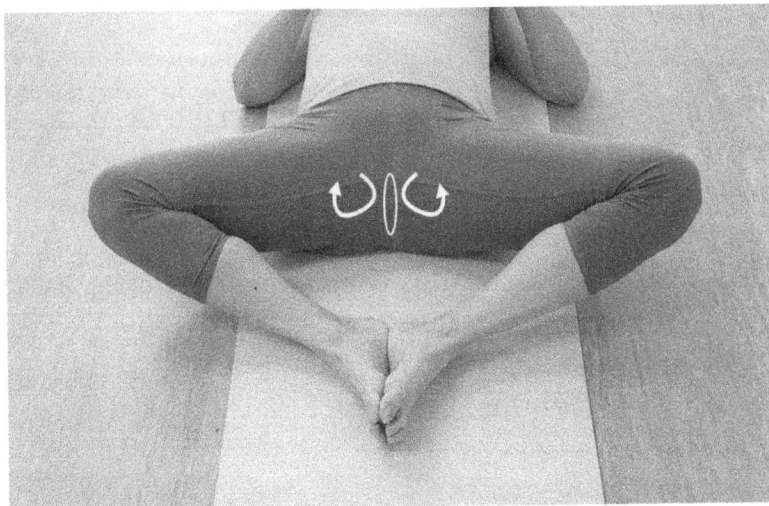

(Image 26)

4. Effleurage on labia lips: This space is not very big; it may be best to use two fingers, or a finger and the thumb. The pressure is very light and is only about the weight of 1 apple or 1 pound. With a little Arnica ointment do small gently right along your Labia lips right and left. Using your fingers and thumb gently apply light pressure to either side of your labia lips. This will feel surprisingly good. Repeat this three times. (Image 27)

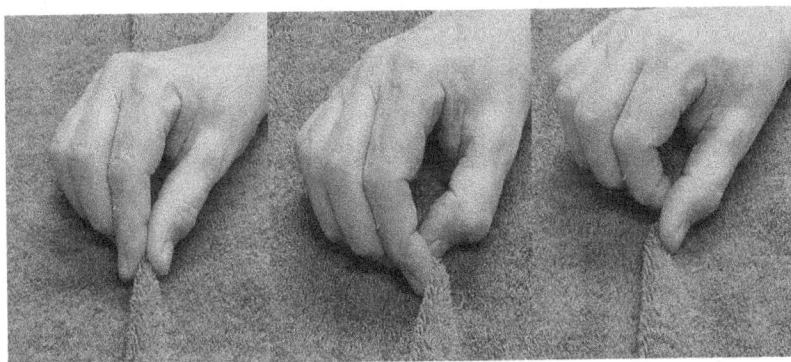

(Image 27)

Acupressure

There are some influential acupoints right along the superior aspect of the pubic symphysis. Those first six weeks, you are too swollen to have done these. It is never good to do acupressure directly near a wound site so soon after surgery. The acupressure points for this chapter are on the pelvis and foot. The points on the pelvis are Stomach 30 *Rushing Qi*, Kidney #11 *Pubic Bone* and Ren #2 *Curve Bone*. You may notice, the points on top of the mons pubis will appreciate the pressure on them.

For these points on the pelvis, expect this tissue to still be tender. Using light, gentle pressure is key to success. Do not worry if you are not on the exact acupressure point; if you are close, that is important. If at any point one of these areas hurts, lessen the pressure and just lay the palm of your hand on the area. Find what works for you. During this time period, this area cannot take too much pressure, so I would lay my hand on the abdomen. Each one of these acupoints Ren 2, KD 11, and ST-30 are great acupressure points to help bring healing and Qi to the area. I generally wait between week eight to10 to directly needle these points in my professional practice as there are just so many other ways to influence the vagina with distal acupoints on the feet, head and hands. Pressure should be the weight of one orange, or one pound. If you feel you can take more pressure, this <u>DOES NOT</u> indicate you can add five pounds of oranges of pressure.

Pelvic Acupressure

Ren-2: *Curved Bone*. This point is the second point on the Conception channel or meridian. The name pertains to the natural curve of the bone at this point of the pelvis. Be gentle. Place your finger on your belly button, and slowly slide it down until you come to the top of your pubic symphysis. This point is right on or above the suspensory ligament where your clitoris is attached. You will find just resting your index or middle finger on the area is enough. You can do small circles on this acupoint (Image 28).

The Kidney acupoint is on either side of Ren-2. KD-11 *Pubic Bone*, this point is 11 of 14 points on the Kidney channel. This point harmonizes the lower belly and also pelvic cavity. It also influences and nourishes your body's vital essence. This point is one thumb-width away from Ren-2 on the Ilium bone, on either side of the pubic symphysis. Stimulating this point will benefit Qi flow into your new vagina (Image 28).

ST-30: *Rushing Qi,* Stomach meridian. This point regulates Qi in the lower belly; it also brings balance to the abdomen and core Qi of the body. This point is just lateral to the Ren 2 point. As a young acupressurist I learned this point 20 plus years ago early in my studies of Chinese medicine and I have appreciated the benefits of this point ever since. Use light finger pressure in the area. Do slow small clockwise circles, or just hold this point for 2 minutes. To locate this point, use the index or middle finger of each hand to find ren 2. Slide to the side about 2 inches (5 centimeters), away from the center of the body, to find this spot (Image 28). Two hands are better than one, so using one hand on each side, apply pressure to each side simultaneously. While working along the front of the pelvis you may find a small mass of tissue under the skin. Do not apply too much pressure to this area. Be gentle and respectful of your body around this part of the pelvis. It will still be sensitive and inflamed.

Phantom Sensations

During these initial weeks of healing, there have been a lot of nerves reconnecting to new locations. These new locations can be a little confusing for the brain during the first few months.

You will most likely have experienced a nerve zinger or two by this point in your recovery, which is a good sign. Going back to work will increase demands on your body, which will bring new awareness to your new vagina and genitals. One part of this awareness may be phantom sensations. Most often, this will appear as a crushed or a "racked" testicle sensation. This is an uncomfortable sensation to say the least. As stated before, consult your physician if these are not lessening and use your prescribed NSAID's (ibuprofen), as they have been shown to help with that inflammation.

There are a few other parts to these sensations too. You may have a sensation of an itchy testicle, but on the inside. This, too, is annoying and may lead to some dysphoria. Please look upon these sensations as a good omen; the nerves are reconnecting and transmitting their awareness to the brain. That sensation will be replaced by a realistic version of your genitalia in time if it has not been already. If you itch it, the dysphoria will generally ease.

As for "phantom limb pain," I have known very few individuals that have ever felt such a thing when it comes to the penis. This is not to say it is not out there. Initially out of surgery, it felt like someone had sewn right through the head of my former penis. That sensation went away after the first 24 to 48 hours. Then, around nine weeks out, it felt like someone was stretching the top of my former appendage across 100 yards. That was a good example of when you may need something to break through that pain. Not one over-the-counter medication is working at taking that particular sensation away, so I ended up taking one of my stronger medications, and that took the feeling away swiftly, and it never returned. There are a few patients I have treated for whom stronger medications were not successful at easing this sensation, and there was some residual pain that mimicked the former appendage and/or a crushed testicle. This is where acupuncture has been shown to be very effective. If you are experiencing this sort of pain and medications are not resolving the problem, please seek out an acupuncturist who may be able to resolve these sensations.

Phantom Personal Note: At one point on a weekend afternoon during this particular recovery phase, I could not stop this one annoying sensation. It felt like sweat was running down one of my nonexistent testicles. I spent the next hour or two not wanting to touch the spot. I did not want to validate this dysphoric feeling. The sensation was acutely dysphoric for me. Finally, I did reach down there to provide a little relief to the itch; my finger slid right into my vagina. Not what I was expecting! I could not stop laughing. The sensation was immediately resolved, and dysphoria slid away. Personally and professionally, I have seen this in a few different aspects. One primary point that I proved to myself was that I did not have a testicle! Woohoo. Secondly, the itch went away, and the sensation disappeared, YAY. Thirdly, and most importantly, the nerves to the graft were healing well. Because if I am having that sensation, then the nerves into the vaginal wall are recovering well. This only happened twice. After confiding this to an AFAB friend, she shrugged and said, "You know, sometimes the AFAB vagina itches, too."

Nourishing Nuggets

Discharge: your vagina has been learning these last six weeks, and some non-mucus tissue is educating itself to a new environment. This tissue has been slowly adapting to its new internal setting. With your consistent twice daily dilation, and even with a douche afterwards, you may still have discharge because of the natural cavity of your vagina. Have a few of your favorite pads in your bag or purse to use throughout the day.

Changing your pads regularly will feel good and will also decrease a risk of a rash or fungal itch issues.

Perineum: this space between the rear of your vagina and the anus will remain sore and swollen during these few months. It may feel irritated because it, too, is a part of the surgical site. Not only is it sensitive and full of nerves but there are also sutures in the area, too. Expect this area to be swollen and irritated for the time being. In Chapter 7, we will cover more on the care and massage for that area.

Under the Skin and Nerve Sensations: when giving yourself a self-massage around the lower abdomen, you may find some ropey tissue under the skin. It may be near one of your lateral suture lines used to stabilize the upper aspect of your genitals and vagina. Remember the sutures around the vulva and clitoris are powerful and thick. I cannot emphasize enough that there is a tremendous amount of tension that is held there. You may at times feel there is something under the skin or have a mild burning nerve sensation in the area. Continue your massage work in the area; it will dissipate in time. Apply arnica ointment or gel. You will want to consult your physician to find a prescription to ease any continued discomfort.

Clothing: you may find wearing tight clothing such as jeans or leggings may be a little uncomfortable. This was a bummer for me because I had always been self-conscious about wearing leggings while in a tuck, and I was very excited to wear them now that I didn't have to worry about that. However, the tension and pressure of the tight clothes after a few minutes caused some pain in or around the surgical site. These sensations and issues lessen after the 12 to 15 weeks timeframe. So be patient; those clothes will be super comfortable soon enough.

Cushion: your donut or neck cushion will be seeing a lot of use during these weeks, and maybe for some time after this as well. You may want to get two because, inevitably, you will forget one of them at work or home, and then there is the chance that one of them will develop a leak. This time period is also when you have the risk of overdependence on the cushion, which can lead to reduced blood flow into the surgical site. The skin will become leathery and tough, and this could lead to some dysphoric feelings. Keep an eye on your pelvic floor and the tissue surrounding the new vagina. If the skin down there becomes overly hard or tough, get in there with some self-massage to break up that hardened tissue.

Micro-orgasms: some individuals have experience with this during dilation. It is subtle. However, you may find yourself getting wet from dilation and or from seeing something that arouses you. This is a great start to fuller, larger orgasms. However, it is not suggested that you masterbate until week 12, so please wait to really explore this new sensation. This does not mean you cannot have sexual thoughts, fantasies, or feelings. Just know that the tissues themselves are still in the process of healing and getting rid of swelling. Applying some light pressure will ease some of the swollen sensations to your clitorial area, or a hot compress will help, too.

Chapter 8

Weeks 10 Through 12

Helping other individuals with their own healing often gives you a perspective when it comes to your own. Being back at work had come with some complications and setbacks to my recovery. Acupuncture, massage therapy, reflexology, and Chinese herbs had a profound influence on healing, but they cannot hold back the tide when it comes to the demand we place upon ourselves and on our pelvis during this time period. I was back to seeing patients two thirds of the week while slowly getting back to teaching my weekly dance classes. Giiiiiiirl, I learned that when you teach a ballet and/or dance class, you become intensely aware of how much work the pelvic floor does and how much it has been altered. I immediately noticed when I returned to teaching the limited range of motion I had when bending over at the waist. My flexibility was almost completely gone. It was concerning to me, but I reminded myself that recovery would take up to a year.

Dilating after just one class was enough for me to spend 20 minutes learning how to release and relax my pelvic floor. This is why there is so much written on pre-op and post-op stretching. Generally, the pain is the worst during those initial few minutes of dilating. Give the lidocaine a few minutes to numb the area before starting the dilation. Personally, I was on my feet for 90 minutes when I taught—add to that a 25-minute commute home. I could only imagine what others are going through. I knew I wasn't alone. I charged myself to find ways to dilate in less pain. Take your time; go at your own pace and do not feel pressured, was my motto to start. I began to find that a little massage near the vaginal opening would ease the daily pelvic floor swelling and tension.

I also began to feel some other interesting things happening within my mind around my gender. Explaining it to my partner, I described it as an increased feeling of gender fluidity. I felt my skin's sublayers were a mixture of gender chemicals. At times I would say it was a nonbinary sensation, but upon riding through these sensations throughout these next few weeks, I came to define these feelings as more bigender. I never once looked upon these sensations and feelings as bad. I saw it as part of gender evolution within my own psyche. This far into my transition, the impression of this queer sensation was profound, to say the least. It was as though I was floating on a cloud between these two genders. The best thing I could do was just lean into these sensations and listen to what my mind and body were experiencing.

Healing Weeks Seven Through Nine

At this point, most of the healing is felt internally; the region around the mons pubis, vulva, clitoris and pelvic floor will remain swollen most often due to gravity and the demand you might be placing on your body. If you have the ability to stay home longer, you will find your recovery to be easier than those jumping back into work—but most of us need to go back to work. For me, there was a mounting euphoria during these weeks, and it felt amazing. It was as if I had finished putting the last piece of an enormous life-size jigsaw puzzle into place. You should step back and look at the hard work you put into getting to this point and congratulate yourself for making it this far.

The limited range of motion when bending at the waist will become more noticeable as you increase your activities these next two months. At the start of these three weeks, bend only as far as you can until the surgical site stops you! Your body will inform you as to what your range of motion is. Do not push past that physical stopping point. If you are bending over too far or try to lift something too heavy, the action will make you feel like you might tear a stitch. Knowing when to rest or stop is vital during this time period.

I purchased my first yoga blocks about three months prior to surgery for the dance studio, and they turned out to be very useful in my healing. In fact, the use of yoga blocks dominated my recovery during these weeks. Whenever you feel your vagina swelling and filling with blood, or if there is a sensation of tension around your pelvis, take a break in the next few minutes, and elevate your pelvis on one of these blocks or a pillow if you can. You can work through it and ease the discomfort with a few ibuprofen or acetaminophen, but time off your feet and pelvis will feel great. If you have the privacy of placing an ice pack on your genitals, that will help as well.

Nerves Within Sutures

I once read there were over 150 sutures used in this procedure. You have felt them poke and rub you in just the wrong way during the first six weeks. You have seen them come out in your sitz baths or in your pads. I have also mentioned the sutures at the top of your clitoris and vulva are very thick and strong. If there is a nerve caught up in a suture, it might be anywhere within the surgical site. The consequence of a caught suture can be agonizing, particularly when it involves highly sensitive tissue. You might not have experienced this, and I am thankful for all the folx who do not feel it. However, if and when you get a nerve caught in some sutures, use all the tools in your purse. Elevate your pelvis, and apply ice for 15 minutes while in that position. Apply light continuous pressure to the area; use a hot compress afterwards, and get your rest. If need be, take some

156

prescription pain meds. What seems to be the best approach is to get your self-massaging fingers to the offending location and apply light pressure to soothe that irritation away. If this pain persists, consult your surgeon or your primary physician.

Scars, Scar Tissue, and Nerves

Oftentimes if a surgery is in a particular area, a good surgeon will follow the natural contour and creases of the body. In your case, when creating the surgical incisions for this surgery, the surgeon will follow the natural contours of your body, and in time, this will hide the scars. Because of their location in the groin, some individuals have reported that the elastic from the underwear has irritated a suture line. Trying underwear with thinner elastic around the leg openings, underwear that is looser or a lower cut around the legs, can be helpful. Wearing jeans or thicker material that gathers or bunches up at the groin when you sit may also initially irritate this area. Try to experiment with your clothing at this point to find what is comfortable. For me, skirts and dresses worked well to avoid this problem.

Around this time you may try using a scar ointment on the most lateral scars, the ones located nearest the groin crease (Image 8, Chapter 3). There are some great ways to treat scars. Professionally, I have used a Chinese moxibustion technique to reduce scars in my trans masc patients who have had top surgery. I use a slightly different technique on trans femme scars due to the location and sensitive tissue. When researching scar care, the common advice to reduce external scarring includes the application of antibacterial ointment to keep the skin moist (Padsicles), changing bandages daily to keep the area clean (sitz bath, fresh pads and clean underwear). Avoid scab picking, and reduce any sun exposure.

In spite of these precautions, scarring is generally unpredictable. In your case there are many scar creams and ointments on the market, all profess to remove scars. I would choose one that is organic and all natural. Organic products are grown without pesticides, herbicides, or fertilizers. Although a product may have a "Natural" label, that does not mean it is organic. Look closely at the labels. One old suggestion is the application of a little natural vitamin E oil directly to the scar area. This is mostly anecdotal. However if you want to give it a try, organic vitamin E can be easy to find at a natural grocery store. Take one capsule, and just poke a hole in it to apply some drops to the area. Do this for three weeks every other day to minimize external scars.

After doing some of my own anecdotal research, I decided to use Force of Nature Organic Scar Solution. They have a variety of applications, and it noticeably helped within two weeks. I found this easier to use than Vitamin E capsules, just out of sheer effortless application. If you are concerned about your scars or would like to minimize them, then you will need to carve out some time to dedicate to treating them. It is important to let the scar ointment dry and air out for 20 minutes, so it can do its job. You will want to find the time that is suitable for you; it does not have to be every day. Feel free to spread it out over the course of a few weeks or months. You will see noticeable changes in the scar tissue within a few weeks.

Now only if there was something for these darn nerve zingers. During this time, I personally experienced an uptick in the number of nerve zingers I was feeling–often in all sorts of places. Thankfully, these zingers' lifespan is short and to the point.You will be happy to know these zingers become less frequent in the coming months. Nerves often respond well to heat, so applying a hot compress for 10 minutes has noticeable benefits. If these zingers interrupt your day on a continuous basis along with some other unpleasant sensations, consult your physician.

Dilation

If you are not interested in increasing your width, that is OK. You are not alone in the pain, burning, and tenderness of dilation. The presence of pain is a reminder of recent surgery as well as having a new vagina, so try to focus on the fact that you finally have the anatomy you always wanted. The relocated tissue is naturally tender after surgery, and in some ways, we are traumatizing it every time you dilate. You will see in the end it will be worth it. In an effort to get my point across, I will be repeating myself. The reason it is so uncomfortable is because the nerves in the graft are healthy. Those healthy nerves take a substantial amount of dilation trauma during the weeks and months following surgery. It is also the surrounding pelvic wall that is irritated, which will be causing some of the pain too. But you will only get the depth and width that you want through persistent dilation.

On top of the initial surgery, dilation has to be the second-most painful part of this procedure. The schedule will not relent for the first nine months. If it helps to have some light at the end of the tunnel, between the fourth and fifth month, it stops being painful—or it did for me and many of the girls that I know. Take that breath in, and let it out. There is a time in the coming months where it will not hurt at all. And that moment will be very liberating. I found that stretching my adductors and opening my pelvic floor prior to applying the lidocaine was an added layer of care that helped make it more bearable.

Increasing dilator size is arduous at this point. During weeks seven through nine, you may find having a prescription for some muscle relaxant can be handy too. When you are increasing the size of dilators used, I strongly suggest using the largest one last, and only for six minutes. By then, I figured the lidocaine would have passed through the superficial tissue of the vagina and numbed some of the pelvic floor muscles. I don't know if it always did, but psychologically, it helped to think it did.

There is one other way you can help yourself; your rectal muscle has the ability to tilt the anus in two directions. As mentioned previously, prior to dilation, make sure to empty your bowels and bladder before laying down for your session. Warm your pelvic cavity up with a few pre-dilation pelvic openers and pelvic tilts as shown in Chapter 3. These pre-dilation movements help to loosen up your pelvic floor. Utilizing the blooming flower image as you move throughout your pre-dilation stretching routine can be tremendously helpful, as visualization has been shown to have positive results.

Massage Therapy, Self-Care and More R.I.C.E.

With the return to work, people often have limited time for self-massage therapy. Using what you have learned here and applying just a few things each week will have substantial positive effects, so please do what you can. Maybe your inner thighs do not need the work, just the space around the vaginal opening. During these three weeks, massage around and on the labia lips to ensure they are soft and pliable, rather than sites of gathering fluid. Around this time, someone had given me a gift of a one-hour massage from a transgender massage therapist whom I had seen before. I asked them to be gentle and use little pressure. I was surprised being nine weeks out from surgery just how tender my thighs, gluteal muscles, and hips still were. They were definitely still holding some surgical tension and trauma.

Even with my regular self-massage, the surgical trauma that still lived in my tissues had not completely left.

At this point, besides medications, you have a few tools to help you with post-op pain. Let us take stock of some of the ways these methods may help you in these next few weeks. If you are dilating three times a day, you will find that after a good night's sleep, morning dilations are tender but nowhere as painful as your evening sessions. Your morning dilation could include some light massage of the upper inner thighs and abdomen. Or mix it up with some light acupressure for two minutes on your wrist (LU-7) and hand (SI-3) acupoint prior to dilation (see Image 18 & 19, Chapter 4). If you prefer to stretch or do some yoga before dilating, that would be super helpful, too.

Once you get up and move, your pelvic floor muscles are in immediate use. Your afternoon or evening session might be focused on stretching your inner thighs, or putting your pelvis above your heart with a pillow or yoga block to help drain the blood away from the area. You could gently add pressure and a hot compress to the vulva and mons pubis. A great evening stretch is to take one knee and pull it towards your chest to stretch the iliopsoas. This muscle is tight on nearly everyone in one way or another.

You might have noticed by using the stretching, acupressure, and massage tools in the earlier chapters that they will give you an arsenal of self-care you did not have before. You can also use some cooling ice, or a little massaging directly around the vaginal opening. Listen to your body, and learn what will feel best.

Rectal Issues

During this surgery, they got very close to your rectal wall. The rectum is the last segment of your large intestine just before your body evacuates the bowel. Some of you may have felt it earlier, some not at all. That being said, there may be some rectal discomfort or irritation. There may be issues with continued loose stools or an itchy bum a few months post-op. It could also be an issue of colitis or hemorrhoids. The internal aspect of your vagina came through your pelvic floor and was placed between the rectum and the bladder as in natal females. This is why it is also important to relieve your bowels and bladder prior to dilating.

There is one more area that needs to be covered in the self-massage arena: the perineum. The perineum is the space between the posterior aspect of your vagina and the anus. This area will be swollen since post-op due to the close proximity of your new vagina and your anus. Getting to this area earlier can be precarious. *It was not until these weeks that I began to address it myself. It is not that I did not wish to address the area; it just felt too sore, tender, and swollen those first six weeks.*

It is important to keep the area clean. As discussed earlier, fecal matter is not something you want in a wound. Now that those initial six weeks have passed, and the risk of infection has decreased, you can begin to address this area. Using a little arnica ointment, apply light, continuous pressure (weight of one orange) on the perineum area (the area between the vaginal opening and the anus). Hold for 30 seconds; then let it go, repeat three or four times. This area will still be tender and swollen, particularly if you are working full-time, and getting off your feet will be helpful.

As a former massage therapist and someone who has spent countless hours in physical therapy from my numerous dancing injuries, I do not think you will find that many massage therapists willing to massage around your new genitalia. This is one of the primary reasons I gave you, the reader, so much instruction with pictures and massage tools. Pelvic floor specialists and some physical therapists who are trained in pelvic floor therapy and rehabilitation are amazing, but they are not always easy to find. These individuals are more prepared to get all up in your private areas.

As mentioned in Chapter 1, researching a few pelvic floor physical therapists prior to your surgery will help you. Set up a consultation, and if you like them, make a few appointments with them. These people can be very helpful, even critical, especially if the clinic is not providing one for you.

Now, when it comes to insurance, you will want to have your doctor suggest at least 15 to 20 physical therapy treatments. It will always be better to have them prescribed by the doctor than just asking or expecting it to be part of your insurance policy. If you cannot do that, then you will want to ask how many PT sessions you are allotted. The best way to guarantee a good amount of therapy sessions would be to have your primary care doctor write a script for added physical therapy sessions. Please understand these sessions do not mean your PT will be dilating for you. It is for you to learn how to release the pelvic floor and to establish pelvic floor awareness. If you do not have the access, you may want to review the massage lessons throughout this book; it will go a long way in your recovery.

Decreased Dysphoria

For many individuals, there will be a continued sensation of pulling and swelling around the mons pubis, pubic symphysis, and vulva for the next few months. This awareness and sensitivity may lead to some general dysphoria despite the visual and mental euphoria. It will subside a little with simple self-massage, stretching, and keeping (or getting) off your feet. Professionally, there have been some patients who come to me to ease this sensation. If you want to know my secret, I will often use some of the exact same acupoints I have given you here in this book.

Around now, your vagina and vulva will have noticeable improvements. One of these upgrades is how your surgeons attached your clitoris to the suspensory ligament. In our case, the suspensory ligament is what held your former appendage in towards your body. It is attached to the pubic symphysis. This is the ligament they have used to attach your clitoris. Due to the nerve innervation, sensitivity, and swelling, it will still take some time to heal that region. A hot compress is wonderful on your clitoris. It was about now when I began to test this ligament out. One way to access this ligament is when an individual wants to stop their flow of urine and retract their bladder. This action will pull up on your clitoris. Some of you may actually feel your clitoris tug upward. I think this is an ingenious facet of this procedure. Around now is when I got up in that area to apply some arnica ointment. If your wounds are closed, at this point you can apply a little arnica ointment or gel to the clitorial area to ease inflammation.

Nourishing Nuggets

An Itch: One day, a patient came to me with the symptoms of an unrelenting rash around the sides of their vagina. They had tried basic organic powders, medicated powders, balms, Vaseline, and creams. Nothing seemed to help this individual. Their internet searches suggested neuralgia and an aggravated nerve. Upon some more extensive questioning and examination, we came to the conclusion that it was fungal itch. Two consecutive weeks of jock itch cream alleviated the discomfort. We also addressed a better post-urination wiping technique. It turned out some residual urine was irritating her skin.

Dilation Management and Secrets: There will come a time when you step up from the number one dilator up to the number two size. It was around week nine that using the number one dilator became ridiculously easy, so I began my physical therapy with the number two dilator and skipped over number one altogether. I did this for three or four more months going forward. Just using the number two and three dilator sizes for 20 minutes, I never lost depth. To me, if number one and two hurt just the same, even with the use of lidocaine ointment, why not just use number two and three?

How you manage your physical therapy is up to you. Dilate longer, and you may develop an irritated pelvic floor. Dilating with just small dilators will make penetrative sex hurt. Once I tried the number four dilator, the pain was widespread. Practicing just five minutes twice a day with number four for one month made penetrative sex easier and less painful. Dilating with just the number three and four will hurt for a long while; however, it will make penetrative sex much easier.

Professional Notes*: I had an individual come into my office at 10 weeks with recurring painful sensation. Studiously I dug into acupoints and techniques to assist this patient. This particular patient was also afraid of lots of needles. In my years of research, I came to find copious ways that acupuncture can benefit with just a few acupoints. This time, I was not surprised when she got off the treatment table and said, "I no longer have that pain." We scheduled a second appointment.*

Upon her return two weeks later, she confided to me that since the last session, she had no recurring pains. Much like those trans masc individuals seeking scar reduction, it just took two sessions for this individual to completely eliminate her residual post-op issues.

Chapter 9

Month Four through Six

Throughout my recovery, many of my trans friends kept telling me that things would change during this next year. They didn't always elaborate on what those things were, though, so I was not sure what to expect. Now I know that there were so many healing changes it would have been hard to list. But I want to share them with you here, as I learned so much during this time period. These months have a lot in common and generally focus on things other than wound care—which is really nice at this point.

One nice aspect of recovery is being able to slowly eliminate crutches we have used up to this point. There was a patient and friend who told me that around week 11 she stopped using the donut cushion. Like always, I will say do what is good for you. I did start to slowly wean myself off of it during weeks 11, 12, and 13. There was one thing I had been especially looking forward to—a hot Epsom salt bubble bath. After months of using sitz baths or just letting the water run off my body, I was really looking forward to a deep soak, something that could relax my whole body, rather than just a part at a time.

If you have a bathtub, grab a cup of Epsom salts, some bubble bath, and soak it up. Let that water engulf your body. If you do not have one, try to go over to a friend or family's house to borrow their tub. You will just love that first bath; take a second one, and a third if necessary. And IT IS NECESSARY. If you have access to a swimming pool, go for that long-awaited swim (although make sure your physician gives the OK). Allow that water to wash away the last remaining gender dysphoric mud that is left. It is all about to change.

There are some wonderful bath recipes and bath balms that will ease away your body's tension. If you are going with a premade bath balm, look for the more natural products. I use the old-school recipe of bath bubbles, one and a half cups of unscented Epsom salts, and one cup of apple cider vinegar. If you have the time at the end of your long day to soak before dilating, that would be amazing. I would recommend unscented Epsom salts, as not all the scents put in are completely natural, and some have excessive perfumes and alcohol in them.

Now, when you are in your hot bath, I would also recommend a little light massage around your genitals. This, again, will help any extra fluids trapped in the pelvic area to move out, which will provide relief to you. Epsom salts have been shown to relieve sore and tight muscles, like your pelvic floor in this case. This is why it helps to have that bath before you dilate. As a bonus, it has also shown to help reduce migraines and stabilizes moods. Hot water, soothing Espom salts, maybe some bubbles or bath balms, and some gentle massage will ease the pelvic floor and continue to improve your healing.

It will All Change....

I had heard that from so many post-op patients and friends in the months leading up to my 12 week mark, and I was wondering what they all meant. The evolution of your vagina is about to progress forward even more. What will that look like? But more importantly, what will it feel like?

Here is some of what they meant:

The swelling and inflammation around the labia, vulva, and clitoris is mostly done at this point.

The scar tissue becomes less obvious at this point and begins to be less tender. This leads to an increase in your mobility and bending at the waist or squatting down.

The tension under and around the scars will lessen. The scars around the vaginal opening will decrease mildly between now and six months, and even more between seven and 12 months. Feel free to use natural scar solutions (such as Force of Nature) to help diminish scars. Gently massage on these areas will make them softer and more pliable as well.

The inflammation sensations around the mons pubis substantially these next three months. The sensation of a surgical tuck, and pulling or tugging, will continue to dissipate and generally will be gone by your ninth month.

The nerve damaged tissue will continue to regenerate. I realize not everyone wants to do self-massage. I completely empathize. If you have a numb spot in or around your surgical site, and you do not want to do self-massage, you can avoid it by taking baths with Epsom salts. These areas will start to show some improved regeneration with a regular hot bath because the hot Epsom salt will ease the tissue in the areas, subsequently calming the nerves. These next six months, you will see more sensation coming back than during the first three months. Those pesky nerve zingers will also significantly decrease.

Your clitorial buzzing beehive sensations will continue the march forward. At times it will be less noticeable. Other times it will come out of the blue. One time, my beehive started buzzing and it felt like I had bees in my undies. I had to look down to reassure myself there weren't! Another sensation that may come with this buzzing may be an engorged sensation at times. The increase of blood flowing to the area from your healing beehive will also send blood into your clitoris. You may find yourself a little wet with female ejaculate, too. This is all normal and simply a good sign that things are healing in the right direction.

Your vaginal opening will become increasingly erogenous. As the inflammation continues to recede in these coming months, the skin surrounding your vagina should heal and recover nicely. This recovery consequently comes with increased sensitivity to the area, which hopefully you will experience as erogenous. I will cover more on this subject in the orgasm section of this chapter.

Angry Nerves

For some, there may still be some lingering nerve irritation. Most surgeons will address it after the 12-month mark. If you have a caught nerve, it is best to go revisit your surgeon for a consultation. In your case, most revisions around nerve issues are a serious matter. You cannot just go in there and deaden a nerve cluster without knowing the repercussions. You may actually lose nerve sensation into your clitoris. That is not good news. Consulting a surgeon familiar with this procedure is vital. This is a very specialized surgery, and the pudendal nerve group is nothing to tinker around with. Most often these caught nerves will become increasingly angry when the body is tired, or if you have been on your feet for too long, causing excessive blood pooling in your pelvis. Take into consideration that you are still healing.

By the beginning of the fourth month, I noticed an angry nerve right on my right labia lib. The sensation was far from pleasant, but a hot compress always helped. It was consistently in the same spot every time. The nerve felt like a raw, angry string. The burning and pulling of just this one area was so persistent I brought it up to my surgeon. They recommended giving it time. I stayed with ibuprofen to mitigate this weekly issue. *I brought it up to my partner, and he had the nerve to refer me to this book, LMAO. So I did; the next time this pesky nerve showed her head I would get in there with some massage techniques I have used in the past. Not surprisingly, by the end of the fifth month that nerve never showed up again.*

Dysphoria

Do not rule out dysphoria; it may stay around even though you have gone through surgery. I referred to it as "pockets of dysphoria." I would recognize the feeling, and oftentimes I would just have to look down to delegitimize the dysphoria. For others, it will be different, and it is important to recognize it and appreciate all that you have done to your body to make it feel whole. Things might not feel great now, but you are on your way. For me, looking at and touching my body was enough of a euphoric sensation that I could easily dispel the dysphoria.

There is a term I like to use about this time period: "euphoric homeostasis." The body, mind, and spirit connection is profoundly affecting the psychological aspect of your mind. You may be feeling more connected to your body and yourself than you ever have previously. You may actually have felt that awareness earlier than now. The pain of healing can often delay these perceptions. During these next nine months, your euphoric homeostasis will only become brighter and stronger. We will probe deeper into this next subject in the Touch and Play sections of this chapter. The sexual euphoria is philosophically so much deeper—or at least it was for me. No chart or test can measure the acute positive impact of this procedure on your psyche. Gender euphoria is quintessentially enlightening, and I really did have a different perception of myself during this time.

Still Hurts, Swelling Continues to Heal

Yes, you will still have some swelling, and you will still have some range of motion issues, such as bending at the waist. Most noticeable will be the continued tension around the mons pubis and the pubic symphysis. Secondly, the perineum area will also be sensitive and can remain swollen these next few months. The icing on the cake at this point is you can take a bath or hot tub to ease the pelvic floor tension. These two areas will benefit greatly from regular hot baths by increasing blood flow and relaxing the muscles. Stretching helps the areas too, as will gentle self-massage. The donut or neck cushion may be gone, but your pelvic floor will still be healing for another six months. Hard surfaces will not be your friend, so be mindful before plopping down on your hiney these next three or four months.

It will help to fall back to things you have already learned those first three months. If the discomfort is too great, ice will be helpful during this time too. Sometimes, I found that using an ice pack just before dilation to reduce pelvic floor swelling helped. On other days, it was the hot compress, so try to listen to what your body needs. Remember, finding what works for you will be most important. This will also help with the ongoing tension around the mons pubis. If you do not have time for a hot bath, applying a hot compress on the area will calm the strain.

Months Seven through Ten

If you had either a shallow or a full depth procedure, your cardiovascular system took a small hit during this procedure. If you had a semblance of a workout prior to your procedure, this is a good time to ease your way back into it. A mild anatomy lesson may help you. Your hamstrings attach to your pelvis; one head of your quadricep muscles attach to the pelvis, and your adductor muscle group attaches to your pelvis. We must not forget about the big mover and shaker, the iliopsoas, which is also attached to the pelvis. All of these muscles play a huge part not just in your daily movement, but even more so in physical workouts. So you will want to go slow as you ease back into being more active.

Instead of breaking down each individual type of workout, I have grouped them into low-, medium-, and high-impact activities. Going into your workout cautiously with a keen eye on how your pelvis feels is your starting point. Slowly leaning into your workout versus jumping into your prior routine will be a good philosophy. What would leaning into a workout look like? Say, for instance, you had a swimming routine prior to your procedure, and you were used to swimming for, say, 30 minutes for your workout, using various swimming strokes. I would suggest five to 10 minutes of swimming the first time out and reducing the number of strokes you do to those that are gentlest. Over the course of the next two to four weeks, build back up to your former 30 minute workout. As you can see, the pelvis serves as a major hub for muscle attachments, so consider it a bit of a weak point at this stage. Treat it like you would a sprained ankle; go slow to see how much it can tolerate. Before you jump into your workouts, review and break your former routine down into smaller segments. Start slow, and let's review some workouts and potential issues that may arise.

Low Impact

These activities will include walking, Tai Chi, Qigong, gentle yoga, swimming, or golf (sort of). These activities are by far the easiest to get back into moving after your surgery. These movements are slow, controlled, and the requirements on the pelvic floor are moderate. Walking is one of the best exercises to get moving again because it is so easy to moderate your pace. If your pelvis is feeling good, you can easily walk faster or up an incline to expend a bit more effort. I recommend to my patients Tai Chi and or Qigong, which can be very beneficial during the next year. Tai Chi is more of a defensive martial art, while Qigong is a movement that nourishes Qi and cultivates an individual's energy. You can find some restorative Qigong on my YouTube channel: Queer Dance Project QueerDanceProject.com.

If you can find a particularly slow and gentle yoga class, it would be great for your initial foray into moving again. If you previously did yoga, you may have already slowly done some yoga movements, perhaps without even thinking about it, because your body was telling you to stretch and bend. If you don't want to go out to a yoga class just yet, you can find a slow and gentle yoga class to stream on YouTube, iTunes or on a VR device. If you are going into a faster paced yoga class you will run into mobility and range of motion issues the first two months, but it will slowly improve.

Swimming has several strokes including: breaststroke, butterfly, freestyle, and backstroke. Some of these strokes will be easier than others. You may also want to add a side stroke into the mix. The nice thing about swimming is its low-impact nature; your joints are not being impacted nearly as much. The breaststroke will have an impact on your pelvis since the adductor muscle group attaches right next to your new vagina and is heavily used in breaststroke. Although it would be therapeutic for lymph flow and muscle toning, it may be difficult early on. You can adapt this stroke by not using such a wide kick. The butterfly is one stroke that will have an effect on the lower abdomen and your groin area, so maybe leave that stroke for month seven. The kicking motion of the freestyle and backstroke will be easiest to start with. Start slow, and build up your former routine.

Golfing could almost be placed in the medium impact area. There is a great deal of torque and twisting involved with golfing that uses the pelvic muscles. In turn, the strength of your pelvic muscles will also affect your golf swing. Lastly, the speed with which you swing your club requires quick responses from your muscles. You may want to bend your knees to place the ball on the tee rather than bending at the waist. It might be best to test out how your pelvis feels by visiting the driving range first. Take your time, and feel how your body is responding; it will tell you if it is not ready for a full golf game.

Medium Impact

Some examples of medium-impact activities are dancing, running, hiking, and cross-country skiing. Let's talk about each of these. Many types of dancing are low-impact, but there are others that will require more impact such as hip-hop, tap, some jazz, and others. I place dancing here under medium impact because of the high involvement of your pelvic floor. Slow is the way to go with dancing, no matter what type of the art movement you chose. The pelvic floor will be active and functioning a lot, as well as all of the muscle groups in the legs. Start nice and easy, remembering to take breaks and rest when needed, and don't expect to have the same stamina you did before surgery. Remind yourself that bending at the hip will be limited for the next three to five months.

For runners, I would really encourage a warm-up phase, say five to seven minutes of slow to medium pace. This can lead into a light run phase followed by a short walk phase. Listen to your body. The run-walk method is great for just starting out. Jog for 30 seconds walk for 30 seconds, building up over the next coming weeks. This will allow your pelvic muscles to strengthen at a good pace. I would recommend dilating beforehand if you can because your pelvic floor will be irritated afterwards.

Remember, you may have some added discharge as the pelvic floor squeezes out any remaining liquid in your vagina, so wear a pad the first time or two to assess if you need one. Also, replacing your running shoes every 500 miles will be better on your feet, ankles, and knees.

For hikers you will want a low-impact surface in these early months. A level and smooth walking surface is perfect. You can slowly and build up to paths that have steeper inclines and more uneven surfaces over the next three months. Once you start going after steeper gains, your pelvic floor will feel it, along with the tension that is around mons pubis and the clitorial region. The steeper hikes will ask a lot from your pelvic stabilizer muscles and all the muscles that attach to the pelvis. Be conscientious of how long you have been out, and slowly build up to your previous peak climbing levels.

Cross-country skiers may want to have access to well-groomed trails or nordic facilities to gradually get back into their routine. You can also follow the same deliberate phasing in and building up to longer stints as the runners do above. Using skate style skiing will involve more groin and pelvic muscles, so you may want to start off with parallel skiing initially.

Crossfit gyms have become very popular these last two decades. The amount of core and lifting asked of your body during crossfit will definitely place stress on your pelvic area. If you are up to building and strengthening your core, getting a good core routine from your crossfit instructor is a solid place to begin. With the limited range of motion still within your pelvis, bending over may still come with constraint. You may want to wait until week 16 before jumping into your crossfit workouts. That being said, you may be able to mimic the workouts with lesser weight or doing them more slowly.

Climbing is fun and very exhilarating; it, too, may take you more time to work up to. I place it under medium impact because of the amount of lifting of your body, the stretch placed on the groin area for big reaches, and the possibility of impact with the wall or floor. The climbing harness will cause some discomfort along the scar lines, which could contribute to blood pooling, and this may lead to some bedrest or some further down time. You are using your legs and pelvis to a high extent in climbing; this is why you may need some time to work your way back into climbing through one of the other activities mentioned. Check with your surgeon about a good time to get back into the harder climbs.

High Impact

High-impact activities call for more caution with your very new genitals at this point. Contact sports such as hockey, roller derby, flag football, or soccer, just to name a few, should be eased into and put off until six months or so. Roller derby and hockey folx can get back up on your skates and take a few hours each week to lean into your former workout, but don't start with body contact right away. Since these activities have some cardio and running components to them, following the running guide above will be best. You will not break your new genitalia with an impact after 12 weeks, but it can lead to bed rest and a delay in return to your badass sport. Therefore, take some time before you get into full body contact.

Baseball and fast or slow pitch softball are similar to golf in putting a lot of torque and twisting motions on your core and pelvis, either with a throw of the ball or the swing of the bat. A great way to approach this is to go outside and start throwing that ball around. See how your pelvis and vagina feel. Mimicking your batting swing should be done gradually and without too much twisting, wind-up, or weight. The risk of a pitch hitting your crotch is pretty low. Pay attention to the pain of pitching, throwing a ball, or swinging a bat and assess where you are before committing to an entire game. Ice will be your friend at this time, so don't hesitate to use it.

With downhill skiing, as fun as it might be, the risk of being hit by another skier is present. Further, it requires a great deal of pelvic stabilizer muscles. You will most likely want to stay on the green slope those first few runs out. There may be more individuals on those slopes, but the impact from a fall will be decreased in comparison to falling on a blue or black slope.

Horseback riding and bicycling are both activities that should be done in a controlled environment. If you are using a bicycle, having a stationary trainer to use those first few weeks in the saddle will help you ease into it. It is said in the bicycle industry, "It is best to spend money on the things that touch the bike."

I personally got back on my bike around week 15 using a trainer and really good shorts with super thick padding. Starting slow and teaching your body's tissue to sit on such a swollen and sensitive spot takes time. Most of your time those first few weeks will be just getting used to the saddle again rather than riding for any long time periods. If you have a caught nerve, this is where it may show up or irritate it even more. Using a super soft, cushy bike seat will help too. This particular exercise is very hard on the surgical site.

Horse riding may be a little harder than bike riding. You may want to just spend 10 minutes sitting in the saddle for one minute and then standing up in the stirrups for one minute. It will be slow going those first two weeks, but it gets easier. When you get off either the bike or horse saddle, the blood flow into your vagina should feel good, but listen to your body the next day to see how sore you are.

If you are into boxing or if you're a martial art, start with your beginning forms, and build up from there; don't jump into full contact right away. You also may want to limit your high kicks in martial arts initially. When you are in sparring situations, you may want some groin padding.

For the triathlon folks, the trifecta of sports will take time to build back into. Use the swimming, biking, and running information above. Your post-workout care should include elevating and icing your pelvic floor, taking a hot Epsom salts bath, and resting.

The obvious takeaway from any of these workouts is to check in with your body. On those first forays back into doing some sort of activity, pain may show up the following day, so that is why I recommend exercising for shorter amounts of time initially. The fact that you have been resting a lot during the last several weeks also means your cardio will take some time to build back up. Recognizing when to stop and when to push yourself is important. Drink your water in all of these activities, as it will help with moving fluid out of your pelvic area.

Dilation

There is an amazing point to this moment in your recovery. If you have been constant with your dilation practice these last three months, you will only have to dilate twice a day. LET THAT SINK IN. This is a great achievement. You will start to notice that it does not hurt as much, unless, of course, you are moving up in width.

Now let's talk about the depth and width a little more. If you are still working through some discomfort with the largest dilator, don't feel bad; you are not alone. There is some anecdotal evidence from three of my patients that it was the wider larger

179

dilator that helped break into that larger size, which allowed for easier and more enjoyable penetrative sex. One patient used a solid glass dildo, rather than the largest dilator, to ease the dilation pain. This also helped them with some of their penetrative sex pain.

Now is the time to mix it up, honey! If you want to explore with different dilators, go for it. Trying silicone versions or glass versions might be helpful. Keep in mind to check the width of whatever dilator you choose, so you know that you are meeting the suggested widths. I purchased one glass dildo as a gift to myself on my 12-week anniversary. That celebration was fun yet painful. There will still be pain down there, but in the next 40 days, it will lessen noticeably. There will be light bleeding or some pink-tinged fluid when moving up in size or changing to a different style of dilator, as mentioned previously. It is still important to not miss a session—even after a long day on your feet or at work. You are in charge, and you can manage your sessions the way you desire. Make sure those dilators are in for a minimum of 15 minutes to guarantee the greatest results. This part of your healing will be more fun and easier than the last three months. Dilation is reduced; you get to explore new penetrative ideas. If you are looking for something more lifelike, there are a plethora of dildos out there. I might suggest going with something the size of your smallest two dilator sizes. I went too large on one purchase and regretted it. Using the Intimate Rose for penetrative sex was also great practice as well.

When you are on vacation and or visiting someone, dilating and traveling with dilators could be problematic or at least require some creative solutions. When visiting family or friends, the easiest way I found to deal with this was to just say I needed to do some physical therapy and retire to a private area to dilate. We may want to tell—and even yell—that we are dilating because it is such a struggle to get through it. However, other people may

180

think it is a little too much information. Not everyone wants to know every single time you are dilating. Referring to dilation as physical therapy (PT), which it actually is, may give people a more understandable perception of all the work you need to do to recover from this surgery. *But that is just me—You do you.*

If you have to fly while recovering and are still dilating on a daily basis, you might wonder how to deal with the TSA. One individual I knew just told the TSA agent exactly what her dilators were for—They left her alone immediately. Although it is inconvenient, it got to the point. I find the direct approach and/or using humor is the easiest with TSA agents. If I had to travel during this time period, I would bring my dilators in my carry-on luggage. Think of your dilators as medications; you need to use them every day, so bring them with you. Having a response handy if security were to ask about them will be helpful. There was a friend of mine who lost her luggage for her three-day trip, so she just stopped by a porn shop and picked up a few items that would do the job. Eventually she recovered her dilators. Your dilators probably aren't even the most interesting thing they have seen all day. So smile and move on through.

There will come a time when you will want to be done with dilating! Having that discipline and self-respect is within you, though—You can do it! I know a few folx who tried integrating penetrative sex for a dilation session. They ended up having to return to their former dilation routine to prevent a decrease in depth. I would personally not recommend replacing penetrative sex for dilation, nor will your surgeon. I do cover some of that subject below. Remember to breathe, and that you are the manager. Have patience with yourself and if you can move up a size dilator near the end of your session, that will help ease some of the discomfort. I have known some girls who would dilate with two of the smaller ones in the morning and then use all four in the evening. Others choose to only use the largest ones every other day. Choose what works for you, and don't give up on it.

Be nice to yourself and your new vagina. Practice your stretching or massage techniques to help your pelvic floor relax. Even doing just one stretch can help release the pelvic floor and make it more comfortable for you to complete the session. If you dilate in the evening or before bed, it may help to have a fresh pair of undies to change into during the middle of the night. As you relax into sleep, so does your vagina, which may mean some seepage will occur. This can consequently lead to a rash or a persistent itch. Changing your panties in the middle of the night will help things remain dry and clean.

Personal Thoughts; I had reached 12 weeks; this was when the medical community says you can start having penetrative sex. I was still working through regular dilation pain and didn't even want to think about penetrative sex. I was, however, thinking about learning to masturbate and orgasm. I, like many other girls at this point, just wanted to know what it may feel like to climax. Before I explored penetrative sex, I needed to learn to touch my new body.

Touch, Play, Orgasm

For some of you, learning to touch yourself may come as easy as opening your fridge. For others, having to touch yourself when all you have known is the incorrect gender can be more challenging. It can also be intimidating and scary to touch yourself in this manner, as your genitals have been a wound for so long. Find and take the time for this. Turn the lights down low and caress yourself in the morning, in the evening before going to sleep. Practice compassionate self-petting, caressing. This playing breaks down what unseen barriers may remain. These are all ways to breathe into your new body, to feel a different sort of embodiment than you have previously experienced. Those first few times, I giggled constantly; the sensations were mildly similar and yet profoundly different. All I could do was giggle and laugh. It was important to me to erase the recent images of the last three months and create new and bright sensations. Touch is a brilliant way to do just that.

Now for some fun stuff. You may not have this on your radar, but many of us do. Sex and orgasms are not recommended until you hit the three-month mark. This is when the surrounding sutures have largely healed and closed up. At this point, there is one question I hear at my acupuncture practice from post-op patients: when can I touch myself? What will it look like? And how much time should I spend? Much of your superficial healing should be coming along nicely, and touching yourself in a safe way without risk of infection can now begin. This next part is all on your own schedule. Take your time to explore. Do this however you wish; make it something special. Take the time to create, imagine, and envision what this may look like. Turn the lights off; turn on some music; light a candle, and relax. Take the time to caress and explore with your eyes closed. This allows you to settle into your body and really listen to what it is telling you.

This exploration should involve your whole genital area.

For me, I was a little nervous to touch my new genitals in a sexy way. I was increasingly horny, but I was unsure about using my "new equipment." I don't know if I was worried about breaking it, worried about any open wounds, or just afraid because it was so damn expensive! Whatever it was, I had to spend some time with just myself. I had to allow myself a period of slow exploration, of figuring out what felt good, what felt great, and what was too sensitive to touch. I highly recommend taking your time here and doing this by yourself initially. It can be really overwhelming in the sense that you are feeling so much in so many different ways. You are feeling happy about having the correct genitals; you are feeling horny, as you haven't had sex for the last three months; you are worried about touching your new vagina; you are worried about having an orgasm. Your brain will be pulled in many different directions, and that is why I recommend you take some time with yourself to explore over these next few weeks.

There is a huge chasm that we have to step across after this procedure. The precipice is vast, and the steps should be small at first. Having the inherent dysphoria around your gentilia swept away in the matter of hours is incredible. Relearning what feels good is a profound path through your recovery. There was a struggle in me as a healer to find pleasure from a fresh surgical site. Like that athlete returning from a bad injury, finding the trust within yourself to grow past the memory of that wound takes time. Initially, I was very hesitant to play with myself. I knew what it had looked like down there. The memory of the surgical pain was only a few layers below the surface. Learning to move past visual surgical trauma and daily dilation pain into the arena of pleasure is a passage that can be harder than you think. I was excited yet afraid to even try to masterbate; I knew what it looked like down below those first 12 weeks.

Breaking past the engorged clitorial sensation and looking for the pleasure in that feeling may take time. I was never encouraged to masterbate by my doctors or physical therapist. On the other hand, a girlfriend of mine said on social media that her surgeon encouraged her to masterbate often. That makes sense to me, since we are learning to do something different with the anatomy we now have. The first time I tried using a vibrator, I did not have the advice from another friend. When I put that vibe on the full setting, my vagina and clitoris *were not ready for that at all. It was a few days after my first attempt that a girlfriend recommended keeping the vibrator on the lowest setting these first few learning months. In fact, those first few weeks or so, I would often put the vibrators aside and just close my eyes to feel those new beautiful sensations without the agenda of a vibrator. I did this day after day to break through traumatic sensations and into the realm of joy and pleasure.*

There are some of us who are planning on using their vaginas for penetration and some who are not ready for that or don't want it at all. The first few times you do have intercourse, it will hurt in a good way. You will also probably have some blood as you did when increasing dilators. After those first few times, I made sure to take some ibuprofen beforehand. But if you are not ready for it, there is no rush. Find your buzzing clitoris in its little hiding spot. The first few times I did this, I laughed with excitement and wonderment at the sensations. Get some lube, and continue to explore with this added form of sensation. Get yourself to a point where you feel more excited and less surprised to be feeling things in their new arrangement. Spending time before going to bed or early in the morning caressing the area regularly will relieve some of the ancient dysphoria that has been lodged in your body for years. Those numb spots or aggravated nerves should not be on the agenda for this touch and play time. This time is about learning what parts feel good to be caressed and what sort of touch and pressure to use. There is something profound that touching and playing does help with. Slowly it removes an inherent guarding that happens with injuries, surgical sites or wounds. Taking the time to remove that guarding with continued touch and play is vital. This touch and play does not have to be sexual in nature.

Vibrators

The intention of this practice is not about orgasm. It is to use touch to explore new sensations and feelings. Prior to my procedure, it was brought to my attention by the nurse practitioner that a vibrator would be my friend for future orgasms. At week 12, I had some wise words imparted on me by a dear trans girlfriend; she said, "Do not put your vibrator on the highest setting." And so I repeat: <u>DO NOT put your vibe on the fastest/highest setting at first.</u> Work your way up to that setting; for right now, give it some time, and go low and slow. This is not about having an orgasm; I truly mean it.

Orgasm will be covered later. Your priority is to learn about what it feels like to "feel" authentic. This is a nice way to gently break through some extensive dysphoria that lived there. GO SLOW, practice with and without a vibe, practice using different settings on the vibrator, practice with your fingers, practice with different sized dildos (in width and length). Afterall, practice makes perfect. And use lots of lube! Everything's better with lube. Take the time to explore all of your genital area: your clitoris, your labial lips, your vagina.

Place no pressure on yourself whatsoever; just explore and touch. Feel what it's like to be in your genuine body. Your clitoris and vulva will become engorged as blood will rush to the area as it was designed to do. You might feel like you have a little hard-on. There are some individuals that believe this sensation of being engorged is potentially left-over erectile tissue. For some, this is a contentious/testy/antagonistic subject. It could lead to some possible dysphoria. There are some early confusing sensations between the sensation of engorgement of your clitorial area and the old erectile tissue you used to have. Cisgender women's clitorises get engorged with blood during sex and are also made up of some erectile tissue. What you are feeling may be normal, but feel abnormal to you because of your previous history with erectile tissue. Give yourself further time to heal; wait to see what nine months and then 12 months feels like before seeing your surgeon or seeking a second opinion. I remember those first few times I would look down to see if there was something poking out. Much to my delight there was not. There is a section on revisions later in the book.

There is an amazing euphoria to having fulfilling sex in your authentic body, whatever it may look like to you. These first few times you may want to dilate for seven to eight minutes an hour or so prior to penetrative sex. Something to anticipate is, your clitoris will get excited and engorged. It will be wonderful. If using a vibrator, be gentle. You will find your labia lips are sensitive to the vibrator too, especially if you had sensitive tissue in that area prior to surgery. Go gentle these first times with your vagina if you are having penetrative sex. Despite your use of lube, expect to have some light bleeding from the area afterwards if you are practicing penetration. Your vagina will be swollen and hurt in a good way. Your clitoris will have a tremendous amount of blood flow into it, as will your vagina and pelvic floor. After the fun and games are over, you will be sore when dilating your next time. For me, it felt extremely validating. Those first few times, you may not be able to go the distance you are hoping for. Do not worry about it. That vaginal tissue is still sensitive and delicate, but with time, things will become easier.

Something to also consider is to play and touch in a hot bath or hot tub. You may want some of your vibrators to be waterproof for submersible fun. This is a great way to help soothe the pelvic floor and gratify your clitoris with some light touch and gentle playing. Playing in water allows for the touch or vibrations to be felt differently, which may be easier in these first explorations when everything seems to be extra electrified.

I would encourage regular play and exploration time after 12 weeks to get your body used to different types of sensations. Spending the time **feeling** your authentic body in a compassionate way is powerful on so many levels. First and foremost, it helps to break down pre-existing dysphoria. In breaking through this long-held dysphoria that resides in that region of your body, this will consequently lead to a happier and healthier you as you slowly heal from the mental and physical trauma of being in the incorrect body. Have patience; don't place any expectations on yourself or your body.

Orgasm

This is a powerful procedure for so many; it allows you to live in a body that is profoundly true for you. You may be feeling sexier than you have ever felt because everything is congruent now. You may be anxiously awaiting the time when you can express that sexuality through orgasms. You most likely have been feeling it these last few months with a little bit of unexplained moisture in your undies. *I speculate that with the recent surgery around the penile nerve group and the formation of your clitoris, this newly bound surgical tension naturally stimulates an individual to develop a wet spot just from that sensation.*

It is important to not place any expectations on your first orgasm, or, for that matter, upon someone else. Orgasms can take awhile to happen again, and when they do, they won't feel like they used to. I've known a few individuals who have yet to have an orgasm two years post-op. I have also known a few individuals to have an orgasm at three months. Personally, I had my first big one at five months. Prior to exploring your orgasms, you should spend some time exploring, touching, and playing. Be it in bed alone, with someone, or in a hot bubble bath, this touch does help break down fences that have been put up psychologically. Up until now, dysphoria may have held your body hostage, but thoughtful touching and playing prior to focusing on getting your first few orgasms will pay off down the road.

There may be some hurdles you need to overcome before you can really get into playing. First, there can be some mental resistance related to how your vagina looked immediately post-surgery. Having an image of your surgical wounds those first few months may be a little difficult to get over, and this is why touch is so important. You need to take the time to feel that you are OK, that your genitals are part of you, that your wounds are healed, and that you won't break anything down there. Second is the continued pain associated with dilation. Using the previously described touch will teach you to discern the two types of sensation from each other. Sexy sensations may or may not be associated with dilation, but either way, you will find yourself separating the two sensations most of the time as one feels like work and the other feels like play.

Touch and caressing plays an integral part leading into your first orgasm, but to be honest, there is no way to predict when that first orgasm will arrive. Free your mind of your old orgasmic sensations and from old anatomical practices. What felt like a sexy touch in the past may not feel the same post-surgery. This is another reason touch and play are so important, you need to learn what all of the sensations are with your new genitals. This takes time, patience and compassion, but it will have some amazing ripple effects within your mind, body, and soul.

Use your imagination, and visualize your body when you are exploring. For me, my first orgasm came as I envisioned my vagina opening up like a flower with colors and lights pulsing through it. There might be different pictures that you prefer, but you might refrain from imagining things that are particularly male-coded imagery such as fireworks, eruptions, or a shooting gun. Your new orgasms will not feel like your old orgasms, and so new imagery may help you feel these new sensations. If you find yourself getting frustrated with trying to achieve orgasm, it might be time to stop. For me, it helped to have a mindset of edging rather than orgasm; and yes, women edge too. By edging, I mean relaxing into a feeling of, "This feels great but I don't need to get over the top."

For some individuals, the frustration from the lack of orgasm may become tangible. There are a few tools that you can use to help you through some of the frustrating times. Some may not be aware of the fact that this procedure will leave the prostate gland intact. This is a nice little g-spot if you need help in fulfilling orgasms. Using a small rectal stimulator will help reach this erogenous zone. There may also be a change in the way you feel an orgasm. This will vary from person to person, there is more of a pushing sensation with your female orgasms than previously encountered.

Erase anything you may have known about masturbation, and throw it out the window. If there was something that attracted your sexual desire prior to this procedure, you may try going back to that desire to see if you can get to an orgasm. But, you may also need to find new things or pictures using your body (or your body being used) in different ways. Expect it to take longer to get to that orgasm than it took you in the past, at least initially. Have patience and practice with a vibrator regularly. Higher vibrator settings may be too much at first, and you may find too much vibrator use will numb your clitoral area. There is something to be said about practice makes perfect.

Personal Note: My first orgasm came on unexpectedly. I was tired from being up since the crack of dawn working at the grocery store and then at my acupuncture practice. I was near the end of one of my dilation sessions when I became super horny. I did not care if it was the dilator or the fact I had a buzzing beehive in my clitoris, but all of it required my attention. I had learned to have a vibrator handy in my purse for moments like this, and so I put it to good use. Well once I put that vibe to work, the orgasm came quickly and naturally. And it was a long time coming. As I laid there feeling all of the sensations, I closed my eyes and felt like I had a blooming inside me radiating outward from my vagina.

If you have a sexual partner, or a few sexual partners, it will be incredibly important to have open communication around sex these next few months. Sometimes a partner may place an expectation upon you, or even worse, you may have placed an expectation upon yourself, in what sex should look like or how it should be enacted. A penetrative orgasm is not always achievable at first; having that expectation may lead to frustration. In fact, over 75% of cisgender women cannot achieve orgasm through penetration alone. Therefore, you will want to explore things beyond just penetration. If your partner's penis, strap-on, or hand-held dildo is too large, then go slower; use more lube, and use some smaller toys that will help you open up. There is truly no need to endure pain at someone else's cost.

There is a side effect to clitorial play and touch, and this is the engorged, swollen sensation you will feel in and around your clitoris. The sensation will arrive as a mixed bag for many. There will be a feeling of an erection right around your clitoris, but looking down, you will not see one, obviously. This can cause some serious dysphoria–that there is a sense of engorgement or that some erectile tissue was left in place. I did not like the sensation at first. This is a very contentious issue and is not commonly discussed by many surgeons prior to the procedure.

Surgeons may not realize the impact of this particular sensation on trans women. However, cisgender women do have some erectile tissue associated with their clitoris and for this particular procedure to be successful, there is a small amount of erectile tissue left just around the clitoris area and held in place by the suspensory ligament. If done correctly, you can actually pull up on your clitoris by actively trying to lift or move your former appendage. Cisgender women can also do this, but may not be in the practice of doing it. Although this is very hard for you to grasp at first, and frustrating because during these next three months, it will feel like a small erection in and around your clitoris and mons pubis, have patience, and know that it is normal anatomy for a woman. There possibly will be a sensation of being restrained, feeling like your old anatomy is trapped and this perception for some is greatly disturbing. Do your best to breathe through it and understand that while it may feel unusual or disturbing, it is normal for women.

Sometimes I would gaze down there just to visually confirm that I no longer had the incorrect body. Touching yourself to ensure that there is nothing there also helps your mind to understand your different anatomy. Using different forms of our senses (touch and sight) will help your mind adjust more quickly. This feeling will decrease over the next few months, as well as the dysphoria associated with it.

Sexual Orientation and Gender Identity

This is something that is rarely talked about—especially by a surgeon but there can be some fluidity to your sexual orientation after surgery. No matter how you identify sexually there may be changes in you that may not be expected. There can be an extraordinary inner sense or core shift that happens for some people around their queer and/or gender identity during this time. For some, you may find yourself leaning into a more fluid identity. Your mind is having to adjust to a new normal. Your transition seeps in deeper with every passing moment and every new sensation. For some, this enlightenment might bring you to a new sense of self, and some may feel increasingly within a nonbinary spectrum. For me, the best way I can define it was a viscous sensation of gender fluidity.

Initially, at times, I felt neither male or female while having profound nonbinary sensations. You may or may not experience or understand these sensations. For those of you within the nonbinary spectrum, this may actually bring you closer to a part of you that you may never have realized. This newer gender identity may subconsciously awaken something within your sexual orientation. No matter how you identify sexually, allow yourself to welcome some of these new wonderful new sensations. Having these fluid-like sensations within your orientation can be an opportunity to explore yourself more. Smell the flowers, and take the time to investigate these new sensations and feelings. They can be powerful and profound.

For those that identify as asexual, this section may be applicable to you as well, depending on where you fall on the ACE spectrum. Your sexuality may change after you have gone through this procedure. Sexuality can be tied to our embodiment, to the visceral way we feel our body, to the ways we enact and use our bodies. Inhabiting your new body, you may find your sexuality expanding in unexpected ways. For some, you may find yourself being newly attracted to different genders and/or bodies. For others, you may not experience any change, Either way, let yourself feel it and explore it if that happens. Inhabiting a body that is finally congruent with your gender can have profound effects on your sexuality.

Discharge and Irritation

With the creation of your vagina and the rigorous dilating schedule these first few months, there will inevitably be an increase in moisture down there. It can be both very validating and very annoying. A pantyliner will help, as does the cotton crotch in your undies. This continued moisture in your underwear and in the general vicinity can lead to persistent itch or rash. You will want to try and find what works for you; maybe baby powder is all you need, but with the possibility of jock-itch, having some anti-fungal cream or ointment handy will help if the issue arises. Triple Paste diaper rash cream can also be useful in addressing this issue.

Personal note: Between week 10 and 16, I developed a bad skin irritation down there. I tried baby powder, and that worked for a little while, but then it returned with a vengeance. When it persisted, I thought it was neuralgia from an aggravated nerve. Sitz baths and hot baths helped, but the pain became excruciating over time. I tried diaper rash cream and natural salves, but nothing seemed to completely remove the pain or discomfort. It was not until a visit to my primary care physician that we finally nailed the diagnosis. With the excess moisture came some good ole jock-itch. Two weeks of antifungal creams took care of it.

Chapter 10

Seven through Nine Months, Ten through Thirteen And Beyond

Glimpses of Normalcy

There are some wonderful changes these next few months. There will be glimpses of normalcy as you get back to the routine of things. The pulling tension around the mons pubis will slowly decrease, and the tugging will completely disappear by the end of these three months. Dilation becomes super easy if you have maintained a consistent schedule up to now. Any former pain associated with it will just seem to disappear.

Some of that normalcy will be seen with a greater range of motion when bending over at the waist. You will still have some tension there, but it lessens considerably. A mild workout routine will make the tension decrease more quickly. The fullness and swelling around the mons pubis and vulva is nearly gone by the end of the ninth month. Sitting during these next few months will still be a bit uncomfortable, but much better than it has been. The pelvic floor is still recovering, so hard surfaces or long sitting periods will still be troublesome.

As nerves recover and feeling returns to the surgical site, there can be new and different sensations. The way the tissue has been manipulated down there, you may have a feeling as though there is a pocket or pouch around your mons pubis. This sensation is just surface nerves reeducating themselves. Massage around the mons pubis and vulva will lessen some of this weird sensation. This area is also where some very small amount of erectile tissue has been retained, which may contribute to this weird sensation. Even this late in your healing, the nerves in this area will still respond well to hot baths and hot compresses. This is particularly after being on your feet all day or having to sit for extended periods of time.

As some parts or life begin to feel ordinary, there are often residual issues that are still present. These can be anything from nerve zingers to suture pain or numbness issues. This is often when I start to see folx in my clinic with one or more of these concerns. Acupuncture has a tool box full of ways to soothe the Qi in and around your new genitals. Traditional Chinese Medicine is well proven in its ability to help heal and treat various ailments. Please be aware that dry needling is NOT Traditional Chinese Medicine, and the theory around dry needling is vastly different from that of classical acupuncture. Dry needling uses muscular trigger points that do not necessarily correspond with traditional acupoints. Seeking out a licensed acupuncturist and having them use proven divergent channel acupoints to ease potential stagnant Qi will oftentimes nullify some of these nagging issues.

Dilation: Celebrate the fact you only have to dilate once a day now!

This is a time to celebrate; you get to decrease your dilation to once a day. What a relief it is to not have to find the time to dilate and worry about that. But for some, it may come with some other difficulties. I personally love camping; well actually, I love glamping (Camping and Glamour = Glamping). I decided to go camping around the time I was eight months into recovery. When I go glamping, I go anywhere from three to five days. And having to dilate while glamping is rough, but I figured out some ways. If you do have trips planned, it is important to include your dilation on a visit or a trip somewhere. During my first camping trip, I skipped a day just before we returned. I was a little nervous that skipping a day would somehow decrease my depth and width. It couldn't have been farther from the truth. I was so surprised at how easy it was to dilate the next day. If you have been persistent in your dilation regimen up to now, missing just one day is not a big issue. However, I would not recommend missing more than two days at this point. Staying on top of your dilation is still a priority and will have great benefits come the next three months.

If it helps to change your perspective a little, you may try dilating for 15 minutes and then using a few vibrators—yes, plural. This has nothing to do with penetrative sex. At this point, dilation has become a monotonous part of your recovery and life. Since the pain of dilating has gone (or at least decreased significantly), you may want to incorporate a little touch and play time at the end of a dilation session. This is a good way to release yourself of gender dysphoria and give yourself a little reward for all of the monotony.

You may want to begin to look at dilation differently, too. You could start to look at dilation as a little errand you need to run, rather than something associated with pain, burning, and inconvenience. This change of perspective will help in the next few months when you eventually reduce your dilation to two to three times a week. Turn your dilation session into what you want it to look like. Up until now, many are held hostage to regimented dilation times. Being able to shape what that may look like is powerful. Take some time to think about it. One fun way is to take a hot bath and dilate afterwards. It makes a nice end to a day. Or do your dilation first, and finish it up with a hot bath and a few new submersible vibrators. The hot bath not only soothes the pelvic floor, but it also calms the tissue around your vagina. Since dilation does not rule your schedule, find what times work for you. It is still not recommended that you replace penetrative sex with dilation at this point. Penetrative sex is not dilation and should not be substituted for dilation at this point.

Douching, Swelling, and a Hot Bath

I am assuming you started douching frequently during those first three months, so now you are an expert. It is very helpful, and it will reduce any smells and odors that may arise, plus make you feel fresh and clean. It is beneficial to douche at least once a week with a diluted vinegar and water solution. A good measurement for douching is one to two tablespoons of vinegar or hydrogen peroxide in six to eight ounces of water. You can also use a drop or two of soap in your douching container. If you do not douche, you will notice a little smell coming from your vagina while going to the bathroom after about seven to 10 days. Douching in the shower is easiest, but you do you. If you have a smell that persists for more than 10 days, consult your physician.

As mentioned earlier, the perineum is still healing. The area will show some noticeable improvement, and the swelling will slowly continue to decrease in these three months. Your go-to for soothing either your perineum, your vagina, or your vulva during these nine months will be your hot Epsom salts bath. If you have been on your feet from work or you have been sitting the whole day, soaking in a hot Epsom salts bath with some nice bubbles will counteract the strain on those areas while up on your feet or on your tuckus all day. A natural bath balm and some candles will do you some good after these last seven months. You may find too many activities will still wear you down, and you may need a day off to recover. Listening to your body is still important, but things should be quieting down a bit.

Touch, Play, and Orgasm

There are a number of layers to touching and playing that leads up to your first orgasm. First, you have lived through seeing your traumatized genitals slowly transform to reflect your identity. Secondly, the self-massage helped begin to break down some stubborn dysphoria during those initial three months. This also helps reinforce that you are in the correct body. Thirdly, you begin to feel your body as your own. Like the layers of an onion remove more of the pre-existing thoughts around your groin region. It does not matter if you are just reading this and thinking, "Oh Snap, I didn't do the self massage those months ago;" there is never a bad time for self-massaging those inner thighs, as well as your labia and vulva region. The multiple layers of trauma can be reduced in your time frame. If you never want to perform self-massage, the trauma may continue to exist, either located in your genitals, or it may find other ways and places to reside within your body.

I say break down those barriers with a cute little vibrator. Using a gentle vibrator setting on previously traumatized tissue is a simple way to remove post surgical mental barriers, images, or sensations. Play and giggle at the same time; it is worth all the time you spent waiting to get it. Replace that former suffering with graceful touching and light play. Practice, practice, practice. There are a lot of new sensations you can do with these genitals; take the time to explore. You will find your dysphoria slipping away completely during those times.

Range of Motion, Cardiovascular, and Nerve Issues

There was a lot covered in previous chapters around working out and the variety of activities that may be considered while recovering. Due to swelling and nerve irritation at the end of a day of work, it might be best to plan your activities at the beginning of your day or on weekends during this period. If you added a light activity as mentioned in the low impact workouts during months four through six, you will find that your range of motion, bending, and squatting has increased these three months. Bending at the waist has become noticeably easier; you will still have some tugging sensations around the front of the pelvis. If you are going to increase your workout to medium impact, or even high impact, do it slowly, and listen to your body. For example; if you have a roller derby match, see how your body is feeling in practices before throwing your weight around. There is no need to hurt yourself for just one match. You want to be there for the next few seasons. Plan ahead as to what you may want your workouts or activities to look like.

During this time of increased activities or workouts, you may begin to feel one particular nerve or an area that is annoyed. There is one patient I worked with that had an irritated nerve right along her labial suture line. It came on at the end of a long day and during bicycle training workouts. Working with that patient, and after a revisit to their physician to ensure nothing was wrong with the surgery, we were able to reduce some of that discomfort through massage, stretching and acupuncture. These next few months, when you massage or touch yourself, take stock of areas that may be more numb than others, or if there is a region where there are unhappy nerves. I am a broken record, but you have had a tremendous amount of nerves rearranged in an area that is highly sensitive. If a particular workout or activity is aggravating an area, you will want to back off that activity for a few weeks until your body recovers a little more. Acupuncture and Traditional Chinese Medicine can do some wonderful things to help alleviate those irritated nerves and help with any numb areas you might have.

There is something I have found in my years treating transgender patients. When treating transgender post-op patients; be they nonbinary, trans-femme, or trans-masc folks, it often takes just two to three treatments to resolve post-operative pain, discomfort, or unusual sensations. Trans surgeries tend to happen in highly innervated areas such as the genitals, breasts, and face. However, acupuncture and Traditional Chinese Medicine can resolve most of these nerve issues. Therefore, if you are still having problems with nerves at this point, please seek the help of an acupuncturist who can help you with these problems.

Ten to Thirteen Months and Beyond

Dilation, Safe Sex, Orgasm, and Psychological Differences.
This is when folks begin to see the light at the end of the tunnel. For once, dilation does not define your time and life anymore. If you have been diligent, it is around the ninth month where you can taper off to two to three times a week of dilation. Trying to remember when you dilated last will be one of the hardest challenges you may have during this time period. It is so freeing to finally not have dilation be the ruler of your days. Congratulate yourself for all those months of dilation; you know how hard it was!

Movement, swelling, and nerve irritation show noticeable improvement, if not being fully resolved. The pocket or pouch sensation around your mons pubis will resolve. Your range of motion is back to normal, and you should now be well on your way back to your normal activities with no limitations. You may still have the occasional phantom itch during these next few months. You will often start to associate them less with their former anatomy and more with an itch on your labia or near your vulva. Other times, an itch will appear, and it will be associated with some moisture down there.

You've read that most natal females do not have an orgasm during penetrative sex, or from penetrative sex alone. It is best to not expect that you will orgasm solely from penetrative sex. This can often be one of the most unrealistic expectations you can place on yourself—ust don't. You have multiple erogenous zones now: your clitoris, labia, vagina, inner thighs and others. Some of you may also be able to use your prostate to reach orgasm, probably along with some vibrators. Using multiple vibrators at the same time may be what it takes to help you reach orgasm. There is no right or wrong way to do this, but it is always helpful to have all the options on the table. For those of you who do not want to explore their body in this way, that is fine, too. It is your body, and you get to decide what to do with it.

Safer Sex in a Healthy Body

It is important to touch on a few things about your new body moving forward. You are finally in the authentic body. Safe, consensual sex with healthy boundaries should take precedence. There is great information for trans folks on the Human Rights Campaign Trans Safer Sex Guide PDF Shagging and mattress dancing have the potential for Sexually Transmitted Infections. STIs are transmitted from one individual to another through sexual contact, blood, front hole, cum/semen, precum, and anal fluids. Keeping your awareness about the possibility of these infections is important to your health. At-risk behavior places us in vulnerable situations; if you suspect possible exposure, seek out local health departments or STI testing sites.

There are two other important things to consider with your new vagina. In general, most men do not carry condoms or lube with them when they seek out sexual contact. I would encourage having a few extra condoms and a small tube of lube with you in case the opportunity arises.

After years of being in the wrong body and struggling with our identity, we may have also developed low self-esteem. This can come into play when participating in sexual behaviors. Low self-esteem may lead you to participate in more high risk behaviors. With at-risk behavior, there is the potential for violence to happen; having the National Domestic Violence number 800-799-7233 handy might help in times of trouble. Please know that you are enough, that you can say no to things you are not comfortable with. You are incredibly strong to get through what you have done for the last few months— Take that strength with you as you move forward.

Chapter 11

Tiers, Friends, and Family

How to deal with all of your friends and family on surgery day? For me, there were quite a few people whom I wanted to let know I had made it through surgery on that first day, but I knew I wouldn't have the energy to let everyone know. So I came up with a system that separated them into groups that would communicate with each other. I developed a three-tier system. For me, I had one person at the top to pass information down about how surgery went. In my case, it was my partner; they made contact with the first and second tiers. Keep your contact list short; you will be able to contact them once you are out of the Post-Op Care Unit.

Tier 1

This level is for your immediate loved ones or closest friends. These friends and loved ones would be contacted by your lead person. On my particular list there were 3 people; these three were contacted once I was safely through the procedure. On my list it was my brother and sister and my biological father.

Tier 2

If you have some friends stepping up, you can ask a tier 1 person to contact all the tier 2 folx. That being said, once you are stable and in your hospital room, you can personally contact tier 2 yourself, but you may not have the energy for everyone on these first couple of days. Consider having your lead follow up with a group text or other messaging. For me, this was my trans family and dear friends.

Tier 3

For those individuals who have a large contact list, you may want to delegate this tier to those that are there for you in spirit. This tier could be reserved for more distant relatives, friends, or acquaintances. These tiers are a simple way to appoint others to assist you. It is important for you to rest these next four weeks.

In the Event

I mentioned it earlier, and I would be remiss not to bring it back up again. Realistically it helps to have things in line just in the event of an emergency. Having a living will and a medical power of attorney drawn up and notarized helps you and your loved ones should anything go amiss.

Allyship and Caretaking

For me, the definition of an "ally" is a person actively supporting individuals from marginalized communities or groups. In this case, allies may be caring for us as we go through this procedure. Hopefully, they are doing so with unconditional kindness and no judgment. So I am writing this as if I was speaking directly to you, as all of the information in this book is beneficial for you as a caretaker. You can help us when we need it the most. Checking in on us when others may not is an extremely kind gesture. Being a caregiver is a taxing job. When it comes to healing and recovery from this procedure, we can use a little help, or maybe even a lot of help depending on which weeks you are with us. Some of us may not even realize we should ask for help because we did not know how hard it would be or are not in the practice of asking for help. There are ways you can assist us with basic comfort care the first few weeks. The first three to seven days are when more serious issues may arise, hence why we are in the hospital for at least three days immediately after surgery and then see the surgeon generally around day seven. In an effort to keep it as simple and uncomplicated as possible, I created a guide for your reference.

Caregiving

As a caregiver, you will need the following attributes: patience, attentiveness, trustworthiness, dependability, supportiveness, compassion, flexibility, enthusiasm, and exceptional communication skills. If you are stepping up as an ally with us during this procedure, please ask yourself this question: Are you doing it because you care and want to help, or are you doing it for the fascination of seeing someone go through this surgery? If the answer is yes, you want to help, then feel free to step forward and ask if your trans friend needs help with their recovery. But if the above qualities are not your forte, then being a caregiver might not be the best way for you to be an ally. Being a caregiver is hard work. You have to deal with a cranky, exhausted person who is in a lot of pain. We are needy people during the first few weeks especially, and we aren't always great at being patient or communicating exactly what we need.

There are a few ways you can compassionately look out for us in the trans community. I had the fortune of having a few individuals wanting to step up those first 14 days. What I found was that too many visitors drained me in ways I did not realize. This happened after the first visit from a trans friend of mine. I became drained and ended up needing a two-hour nap. When they asked again to visit, I politely declined, but I asked if they could bring some food or a meal after week two, which was when my home caregiver headed back to work. Care is based around the individual needs of the person as well as this particular surgery. In this case, it will revolve around ensuring we are using all the tools we have to heal quickly. Initially that will involve eating healthily, taking care of our wounds, and controlling our pain.

Pain medication is important, but there are also acupressure points on the foot and ankle that will help after day 10. Managing pain is always difficult, especially with the addictive nature of narcotic pain killers given after surgery. You and your caregiver need to walk a fine line between controlling the pain with over-the-counter medications and using narcotics to keep pain manageable. Notice I said manageable, rather than remove all pain. You just had a major surgery; it is expected that you will be in some amount of pain, but the trick is to keep it at a tolerable level and not let it get out of control. If your trans friend has a history of addictive behavior or is worried about taking too much pain medication, have an honest and frank conversation before the surgery even happens. It is both important to keep pain at a tolerable level–it actually helps us heal faster–but not take too much pain medication that we get too high. Narcotic addiction is no joke, so just make sure you use it wisely.

Another aspect of caregiving, especially during the first two weeks, is to monitor the surgical area for signs of infection. This can be a delicate issue because it involves the genital area, and neither you nor the trans patient may be excited for you to look at the area. However, precisely because the surgery was on the genitals, it can be hard for the patient to see the area clearly. An infection has a number of symptoms including fever, chills, redness, soreness, and/or swelling in the area of the surgery or wound. Pain or burning sensation when urinating is a sign of a urinary tract infection. Unusual vaginal discharge or excessive bleeding can also be a sign that the wounds are infected. Cross referencing with the variety of symptoms will be very helpful. These symptoms might be challenging, but fever and chills are a good indicator of infection and should be paid high attention to. For me, I was lucky and was told that I could always take a picture of the site in question and send it to the surgical team to see if it was normal healing or if it was something that I needed to go into the office for. You should know if this is an option with the surgical team.

Of course there are a lot of basic things we will need help with, such as helping us empty the foley catheter bag. It is easiest to go to the dollar store, or something similar, before the surgery and buy a large pitcher that you can dedicate to this and then throw away after we are done with the catheter. The nurse will show you how to unclamp the catheter in order to empty the bag and it is very simple to do. Empty it into the pitcher and then empty the pitcher into the toilet and you are good to go.

We won't be doing sitz baths until after we get the packing out, which occurs one week after surgery. We might need some help getting the water ready for this. Using a different pitcher or other container, pour some warm water in, and add either a few drops of soap or apple cider vinegar into the pitcher and gently mix. Put the sitz bath over the toilet with the holes toward the back and pour in the water mixture. Make sure it is not too hot, as we don't want to scald our healing genitals! Afterwards, just empty the sitz into the toilet, and we are good to go.

It is also important that we remain horizontal or in a slight incline while we are resting during those first several days at home. Having a few extra pillows will be important for our comfort. Dedicate one to being under our knees and the others for our head and upper back. We will also want to be using an ice-pack frequently during the first few weeks. Having a reusable one will be the easiest. It is fine to put a thin towel between us and the ice-pack, as we don't want it directly in contact with the skin. I used a kitchen towel and found it worked well. Remind us to remove it after 20 minutes, as we don't want to cause tissue damage or prevent blood flow to the area.

Food, especially during the first two weeks, should be healthy, soothing, and full of fiber. It is highly recommended that our stools be soft during this time period. We do NOT want to be straining ourselves to have a bowel movement. Therefore, soups are a great starting point during this time. The more vegetables the better, both for getting us extra vitamins and minerals, as well as extra fiber. After the first week or two, you can start returning to our normal diet, but I would highly encourage trans folx to make it as full of veggies, fruits, and natural foods as possible. A healthy diet can make substantial differences in how speedy our recovery will be.

There is one aspect of care that we will need a little extra help with and that is emotional and isolation support. Mind you, we may not realize that we need this care at first. In some cases, individuals may not have someone to be there for them. Isolation is a serious issue with trans folx on a good day, let alone when we go in for this procedure. We may not have family or friends to support us and be there to help us, so we may be more socially isolated than normal. Emotionally, there will be tears of joy and tears of grief, and maybe both at the same time. Expect us to be an emotional mess. Being in solitude with those emotions can be difficult. It may be as simple as popping over and saying hello, dropping off some food, texting us a happy GIF, or any other way you want to touch base. You certainly don't have to help us with everything, but there will be several ways you can contribute to our recovery, such as:

- Help with medication: check in with us on our pain levels or if we need refills, make a pharmacy run for us.

- Help organize and clean: Do we need more towels for dilation? Is everything we need within easy reach?

- Help us lift things that are more than 10 lbs.

- Encourage rest: ask how we are sleeping; encourage lots of naps.

- Healthy, healing meals.

- Relaxation and breathing techniques.

- Acupressure points on foot and ankle see chapter 4.

- Help with mail or packages.

- Empty catheter bag.

- Encourage short walks around the apartment or house.

- Encourage some fresh air.

- Help with preparing a sitz bath.

- Help with laundry.

- Preparing ice-packs.

- Prepare Padsicles (see Chapter 2).

- Grocery shopping: pick up or drop off food supplies or help carry in delivered groceries.

- Emotional support.

- Prepare a hot compress.

- Isolation support.

- Help with vitamins and supplements.

- Bring a treat.

- Help getting us to and from medical appointments.

- Flowers or "It's a girl" balloons.

- Wear rainbow or trans colored shirts or jewelry.

- Wash our dilators.

- Wash the dishes.

- Help prevent boredom

Week One and Two

If you are the primary caretaker and staying with us in our abode, I want to break things down a little more for you. If there is a time we need the greatest help, it will be these first two weeks. Days one through three, we are in the hospital. It is not uncommon for us to be in the hospital for up to one week if there are any post-op concerns or complications. Days three through fourteen will be when we will need the most physical assistance. We will need aid with:

- Water: Make sure we are drinking enough fluids.

- Juice will help with rebuilding our electrolytes.

- Meals: Soups are best during this stage. Try to avoid fast foods or food with too much sugar.

- Draining the catheter bag.

- Boredom: Help us break up our bed rest with things that will distract us from the pain but will not be overly taxing as we will tire easily.

- Help getting up and getting down, going for short, slow walks.

- Premake some food.

- Play a game; bring some cards or your favorite movie over.

- Encouraging us to rest and ask how we are sleeping.

- Generally being our go getter. Undoubtedly, as soon as we settle down and get comfortable, we will realize we forgot something. Bringing it to us is so helpful!

Week Three and Four

At this point, we are starting to be up and about more. As we gain our mobility back, we are often caught between wanting to stand, but not wanting to for too long, as it will make our surgery site begin to pool with blood. We are also incredibly tired of sitting and laying down, but that is what our bodies still need. While we can do more for ourselves, this is when it helps to have some friends and family drop you off some food; we can visit people for longer amounts of time, and we are getting seriously bored or antsy. Weeks three and four,we will need aid with:

- Requesting food delivery, setting up a food train with friends and family

- Having someone do the dishes.

- Walks around your apartment, house, or even short ones outside

- Boredom, having some ideas for new activities Friends and family check-in

- Encourage resting

- Let us do the things we can (except lifting heavy things)

- Events that do not require sitting for too long.

- Drive us to appointments

Partnerly and Pet Therapy Advice

If you have a live-in partner able to take the time off to help for these first two weeks (or longer), this can be incredible. If that is not possible, just having someone to swing by those first seven days you are home will help you with your recovery. The peace of mind just having someone there will ease any emotional ups and downs, as well as any sense of isolation. If they are willing to do some light acupressure on the feet, their visit will help you heal more smoothly and quickly. If you have a partner willing to give you a very light massage to your inner thighs it can feel amazing and help with moving fluid out of the area. I would also like to war,n those partners that are squeamish around wounds, blood, and fresh views of surgery. I know of one instance where a partner decided to separate after seeing the surgical site just seven days post-op (I am thinking that there must have been some other issues, too).

I read in a study years ago that showed the amazing benefit of having a pet at home. It showed that people with pets healed at a much faster rate and without as many complications. The unconditional love and support a pet provides is a powerful tool in your personal healing. Feel free to invite people and their pets over if you know the pet is well behaved and won't be jumping on you. If you do not have a pet, or know someone with a pet, there are pet therapy programs around the globe that can help you. Spending some time with a therapy pet can aid you tremendously. One last thing, and I am deadly serious about this. Be kind to those giving you care. The last thing they want is a mean or unruly patient. They are doing their best to help you, so do your best to accept it.

Chapter 12

Time For Tea

You have done it,; you have summited peaks of pain and traveled into valleys of recovery. Any major medical concerns are in the distant past. There are a few things in closing that should be brought forth. It was mentioned earlier in the book that every individual body heals differently, and not everyone is completely healed even after 12 months. In my practice, I have seen issues develop after the one-year mark. Most often, it is around some small skin irritation or some remaining suture line discomfort.

Skin irritation is not uncommon to those individuals who workout or have excess perspiration. Having the appropriate remedy is the key to your success, such as something for diaper rash. Every once in a while, I will have an individual come into my office with some mild internal stitch irritation. Often, it is around the upper suture lines just to the side of the mons pubis. If you can locate the sore spot, a little <u>gentle</u> massage directly on and around the area can ease the discomfort. One particular form of bodywork that I have seen make a noticeable change in my patients is a lymph drainage massage, particularly for those not interested in self-massage therapy. The results from a professional lymph drainage practitioner can have long immediate and lasting effects. This massage will help clear any fluid that has accumulated in the pelvic region, and get things flowing well again. It is like a good oil change for your car.

Most vaginal discharge will have completely halted. Any discharge still occurring should only dampen the cotton swatch in your panties and will be from dilation, penetrative sex, or your personal play time. If you want to continue using pantyliners, that can be useful; otherwise, you can just let the cotton padding in your underwear do it's designed job. If there is more than this small amount of discharge, consider douching more often for a while to see if it clears up. On occasion, you may still have some pink-tinged fluid after penetration play or sex. If there is actual bleeding during penetration, then you may need to go back to dilating more often again or with a larger dilator. It also may be related to granulation, so if it continues or is excessive, I would suggest you schedule an appointment with your doctor about your concerns.

Gratitude Care

You have asked a tremendous amount from your body and its immune system over the last year. Recognize this with small and simple self-care gifts. These symbolic tokens during those first few few weeks and months of our healing can go far in recognizing that we have surpassed a hurtle. One week I bought flowers for my apartment; another I sprung for a Millenium Falcon tee shirt. Of course, jewelry is also a nice option. These souvenirs are commemorative moments of my healing. They can allow you to look back and see the accomplishments even when still suffering the daily pain of dilation and healing. Feel free to scatter these trinkets throughout your recovery as you would like. There are some significant moments that come to mind for me, like the end of day seven, when the packing comes out. Another symbolic moment would be around weeks three and four and again at week six, since you have made it to the top of the peak and have passed the most critical time when you were at risk of infection or complications. This is just one simple way of honoring yourself and what you have gone through and achieved.

This gratitude care does not have to end after week six or 12. You have a year of healing still to come. The time span between month three and six will still be difficult, particularly with an increase in dilation size. Personally, I did not have the money to have an extravagant gift register. One gift was a nice used Tracy Chapman vinyl album I found at a second hand store. Once it was a nice bouquet of flowers, and a candle-lit bubble bath. These little celebrations can have a large impact on you and your recovery, and they do not have to be costly. These distinguishing moments are a way to look back and know you have accomplished something important for your body, mind, and spirit. In many ways, it is a way of thanking your spirit.

Increased Research, Among Other Things...

This surgery is life-saving for many of us. However, the procedure is not perfect, and there are areas where improvements could be made. Now that more doctors and surgeons are doing this work, we hope that more research will be done. For decades, we have been at the mercy of accepting what was offered at face value. I think we are now in a position to start requesting more of our doctors, surgeons and the medical profession in general. That being said, we also need to be arguing for more coverage from our insurance plans.

You have heard me mention the invasiveness of this procedure and the outright pain experienced during those first six months of recovery. For someone who has worked on those who have fallen through the cracks in Western medicine for over 20 years there is one thing that should be addressed. There should be an increased awareness in and around the pelvic floor, including more physical therapy. This is not about helping your dilate; it is about helping you dilate in less pain. The pelvic floor has been split wide open, and some of us receive less than two full hours of physical therapy. If you are able, please consider seeking out a professional physical therapist that specializes in the pelvic floor.

There should be a comprehensive study done on the application of arnica ointments and gels for post-operative bruising and inflammation. I have seen that the use of these ointments and gels reduces inflammation and decreases bruising in several of my own patients. There are two things we could use during those six weeks while laid up. Those of us who have gone through this journey could use as much help as possible. Any research that helps to minimize our pain is a step in the correct direction.

While I'm on the subject of research, it would be remiss of me as an acupuncturist, to not mention the amazing benefits that acupuncture can bring to the table. There are some very influential points, as I mentioned in earlier chapters. The harmony of bringing these two practices together could result in much better outcomes. I have been amazed at how well Traditional Chinese Medicine acupuncture works in particular with this procedure and the associated pain, swelling, and minimizing scarring. How amazing would it be if your nurse practitioner applied battlefield acupuncture right after surgery, which significantly increases the speed of healing. These basic techniques have been proven on the battlefield with our military.

A Solid Team

This particular procedure has been duplicated around the globe, and each clinic will have developed their own team approach. In my particular instance, I was at Denver Health, which has a comprehensive team approach to an individual's care. There was a team of practitioners that all had their hands in my recovery. The surgeon, the nurse practitioner, and the physical therapist all shared notes and communicated with each other, as well as support staff. All of this communication was profoundly reassuring to me.

Whatever your situation is, whether you are having this done through a hospital program or a clinic, inform yourself as to how your team works. The more information you have, the more prepared you will be. All of this information adds up over time and gives you a sense of security around your healing and recovery those first few weeks post-op. Keep in mind these clinics and hospitals have your life in their hands. The more we know about how they care for issues that may arise, the more we can gain confidence that the outcome will only be positive.

Revisions and Locations

After the one-year point is often the time when an individual may consider having a revision done. In general, surgeons do not want to do any revision until after the year mark in order to ensure everything has healed. There are two reasons to seek out a revision. There are a few individuals I know who had a revision at nine months, but those individuals had other underlying health concerns that required a more immediate response. Healing takes time and should not be rushed. This is not to say that if there was an emergency, your surgeon would not perform surgery. If you are considering it as part of your revision, seek out a specialist. This tissue is often directly associated with the pudendal nerve cluster associated with the clitoris. There is a risk of losing clitorial sensation if this tissue is entirely removed. This is a tremendously difficult subject for many, so if you are experiencing it, don't feel like you are alone. Give it time, and let your body settle into itself.

Most natal females who have clitorial arousal will develop an engorged sensation in their clitoris too. To simulate that engorged vulva and clitoris sensation, there is a tiny amount of erectile tissue left. I personally was able to shift my own thinking about this sensation by understanding that natal females have sensations in regards to their genitals, particularly their clitoris. I hope you take the time and do your research before jumping in for a revision in this particular region. Take time to heal and undertake the suggestions here, only because every surgery has the potential for more nerve damage and an increase in scarring. It is important to consider the pros and cons of having a secondary surgery.

It is hard to remain impartial about the results of my own vaginoplasty. So let me preface this first by saying I would always choose to have this procedure done! Period. If I had to go through it again, I would, without hesitation. With that being said, the vagina created may not look as perfect as you may have imagined. And I think it is important that we, as trans women, start having conversations about what these procedures are like and what the results are. This is how we start to encourage doctors and surgeons to change and find ways to improve this procedure.

The two reasons for revisions are for aesthetic reasons or for procedural complications. Those first few months, looking at your vagina can be emotionally difficult. It is a roller coaster because you finally have a vagina and are elated, but aesthetically, your genitals may not match to natal females. The surgeon kept insisting that every vagina is unique and different, and time heals all wounds. In my mind, this does not accurately describe the situation. For those of us who have been around a natal female vagina, you may look down and see that perfect V you needed. At certain times when you look down just below that perfect V, you may be slightly beset by the location of things. At first, I thought my vaginal opening was too far back, and all the trans women I know have said similar things. There is significant distance between where my clitoris is and where my vaginal opening is, much further than in a natal female. As things healed up, this distance started to be more evident.

One night, while discussing this particular chapter with my trans male partner, I said to him, "I think my vaginal opening is in the wrong location."

To which he responded, "I think it is in the correct location; however, your clitoris is higher up than an AFAB." He added, "Every vagina is different." I learned later that he said this in an effort to ease any worries I had about my vagina not looking like a vagina I had hoped for. It does look like a vagina, but there are definite differences between the spacing of my clitoris and vaginal opening. I believe Hilliary Wilson's illustration for the Oregon Health Science University is extremely accurate.

My partner and my surgeon are correct; every vagina is different, unique, and has its own exclusive and beautiful qualities. There are two reasons that would warrant a secondary procedure. One would be that there are medical complications from the initial surgery. The second would be for aesthetic purposes. I personally and professionally argue that aesthetic reasons are just as important as medical complications. Coming directly from the University of California San Francisco Transgender Care website, Dr. Terry Meltzer states:

> "A common outcome of penile inversion vaginoplasty performed in a single stage (a "one-stage" vaginoplasty), with penile skin positioned between scrotal skin, is labia majora that are spaced too far apart. There may also be minimal if any clitoral hooding (except in heavier patients), and the labia minora may be

insufficient after one operation. Although there are different variations of the one-step procedure, it has been the author's experience that these previously mentioned deficiencies are common. This constraint is due to factors inherent to the penile inversion approach and the limitations of the blood supply. From the standing position and with the legs together, most results appear acceptable; however, upon direct examination or intimate view, the deficiencies discussed above will be apparent. In order to adequately address these deficiencies, the author believes that a second operation is required. A secondary labiaplasty provides an opportunity to bring the labia majora closer to the midline in a more anatomically correct location, provide adequate clitoral hooding, and define the labia minora. In addition, there are many variables that can affect healing and the final result. Specifically, this secondary procedure also allows the surgeon to deal with differences in healing, such as revision of the urethra, correction of any vaginal webbing or persistent asymmetries, or revise scars that are unsatisfactory. These revisions will improve functionality and the final outcome for the patient and might not otherwise be addressed."

I may have noticed some location differences, and I knew from internal and external sensations that my clitoris is attached to the suspensory ligament, as it is in natal females. However, AFAB clitorises are generally slightly lower than where mine sits. But every vagina is unique, different, and beautiful. For me personally, there was so much euphoric validation from my procedure for me not to be interested in any revisions. For those seeking care, it is best to get at least two medical options before going through with this delicate process. However, that might not be possible due to availability or distance from a clinic or surgeon. If possible, ask for some photos of post-revision surgeries to ascertain if it will make a difference in your case.

From my understanding, a clitoroplasty does not make the clitoris location different, it creates a cover around the clitoris known as the clitorial hood. Your clitoris will still remain in its little spot. For both the labiaplasty and clitoroplasty revisions, a surgical mesh is often used to make the area aesthetically pleasing. The recovery time will be significantly less than your original vaginoplasty surgery, as all of this work is relatively superficial in comparison to what you originally went through. Occasionally revisions will require a skin graft. It is also important to know where on your body they will harvest that skin and what it will look like when it heals. When I have seen something of this nature done before in my private practice, oftentime it is the area they took the skin graft from that causes the greatest discomfort. You will find that a number of the massage tools provided in this book will help you, if you do choose to seek out a revision.

One reason I bring up the topic of revisions is to ensure you know that it is a possibility after the one-year mark. If you are displeased with your results, I want you to know that there are still options for you. I also think that we, as a community, need to start advocating that a second surgery be the norm for this procedure and that it be covered by our insurance. Not every person may want a revision, but I think it should be an option for each of us to decide.

For me personally, I am happy with what I have because everything works. I can have beautiful orgasms; I have a beautiful "v" between my legs, and it feels right to me. I do wish that I had been more prepared about where things would be located and how different it would be from a natal female's genitals. I believe we should all be better informed about the outcomes before we go under the knife. There needs to be some better preparation and information about this procedure.

Time Off

For those individuals who are seeking out a full depth vaginoplasty I highly recommend you try your best to take eight weeks off. As a small business owner, I am all-too-aware of how difficult this may be. However, the extensive amount of pelvic floor alteration that you go under during this particular procedure is invasive to say the least. These under-recognized muscle groups in the pelvic floor come front and center stage during the first year of healing. These muscle groups influence every aspect of your life, from breathing to standing to sitting to defecating. Keeping your movement to a minimum even if you feel you can do more those first six to eight weeks is crucial. Don't push yourself too hard too soon; otherwise you might go backward in your healing like I did and have to spend an extra week in bed rest.

Close Your Eyes

There was a time after I had my first big orgasm and that I was scared I wouldn't have one again. The mind and ego can play tricks with us throughout this process. Frustration will only become greater the more you focus on it. I know one gal who didn't have regular orgasms, but her underwear would get wet from excitement after just sitting at work. She was still frustrated with the lack of orgasms at six months. I suggested to her to turn on some sexy music and turn the lights off and just touch herself. Sure enough, she had an orgasm within a week or so. Micro-orgasms are orgasms, too; they will eventually guide you to your first big one. Have patience with yourself and how you are recovering. Using multiple vibrators in different locations with your eyes closed and just playing can be deeply satisfying. Just by closing your eyes and exploring yourself personally, the validating euphoria will often guide you to that big bang.

Lastly, your orgasms will feel completely different than anything before, both emotionally and physically. Physically, my clitoris is more sensitive than the surrounding tissue. This is not surprising, since surgeons use part of the penis glans to make the structure of the clitoris. The surrounding tissue above and to the sides are also highly erogenous, which wasn't necessarily something that I was expecting. In short, all of it feels good.

Orgasms will continue to evolve over the next year (or more). You will find new ways to combine all of the erogenous zones you now have. Take time to explore them all. Invest in different sex toys; explore ways to use your body in these new ways. Explore sex with different genders if that is what you desire. You have worked long and hard to get this body; you deserve all the pleasure you want.

Pee in a Cup... REALLY!

While this book does not talk about male privilege as it applies to gender, I will say that natal males have an advantage when it comes to giving a urine sample. I couldn't believe what happened the first time I had to give a urine sample. The question needs to be asked: Who is the nimrod who decided us ladies can urinate into a cup that is 1.5 inches in diameter? SERIOUSLY, I thought it was a joke when I was first asked at 12 months for a urine sample. To the inventors of urine specimen containers, could you please make them a little larger? Seriously! In post-op, the first time they filled my bladder to make sure that there was no stenosis of my ureter, I peed into a basin. I implore you; hospitals, doctor's offices, medical supply stores, to offer women something other than a tiny little cup for us to urinate in. There is nothing like peeing all over your hand to gather an eighth of a cup of urine for your sample. While we are on the glorious page of medical change, how about we rewrite the book on our mammograms? There must be a better way than to smash our breasts in a vice every few years.

Exposure

I know you are proud of your vagina, or at least I hope you feel as euphoric about yours as I did with mine. The power that embraces you as you move forward in your correctly aligned body is amazing. However, I have heard on more than one occasion where post-op individuals wanted to show their new vagina to others! There are places for that, but some of your friends or colleagues may not be as interested in your new vagina as you think. In fact, my trans masc partner eventually stopped going out with me and my girlfriends because all we talked about was vaginas, dilation, sensation, or surgeries. It does get exhausting for others sometimes. You feel correct finally, but it's not like a new car that everyone wants to see. Not everyone wants to hear about your vagina, or your daily dilation, so share with caution.

Closing

This little adventure began with me treating a trans male for their top surgery scars, fresh out of graduate school. The light came on bright as the noonday sun. I knew there were ways to help trans folx with their post-operative healing. By using acupuncture, acupressure, reflexology, and massage, our recoveries can be easier. In time, I developed a solid platform of care that got me to this place. Honestly, the vast majority of my experience has been through a postoperative lens. Over my career in massage and acupuncture, I have had countless people recovering from surgery come into my office. I've seen the progression of hip and knee surgeries over 25 years. I have seen back surgeries become more successful over that same time frame. Wounded veterans with IED wounds, to broken bones, to thyroid problems, there is a good chance I have treated it. All of that experience helped prepare me for what I was about to go through.

During my preoperative months and years, I would surf the internet for advice on this procedure. I would attend pre-op and post-op groups and ask questions. Due to my hands-on medical massage therapy and acupuncture background, I found I needed more detailed information. I was also curious about what other healing modalities could be used. I spent time on YouTube listening to postoperative stories. Still, there seemed to be something missing around healing and recovery.

Prior to writing this book I reached out to more than 20 trans individuals who had gone through this surgery previously. Many of my questions were based on stretching, massage therapy, acupressure, acupuncture, physical therapy, pain relieving ointments– all the things you find in this book. Of those I spoke with, none of them used acupressure, acupuncture, massage, or ointments such as arnica. All followed their prescribed pain medication, and none of them had major complications, although several of them had minor complications. And once again, I found myself seeing things more clearly. There needed to be more information on our recovery and healing. There are some in the transgender community who are so isolated in their healing and recovery. This is one of the reasons that led me to write a book in order to help others going through this incredible procedure.

Some may wonder, did I follow the advice in this book? I did, although I could have used acupuncture from a fellow professional. Sometimes it is hard to get to the correct acupoints by yourself, and I just did not have the money. I did utilize all of the stretching, massage, and acupressure information in this book. I also sought out professional Chinese herbal guidance from my fellow acupuncturist. When talking to the trans women in my life and on those surveys who had gone through this procedure before, none of them had done self-massage, stretching, or acupressure. Anecdotally, when asked how long it took to feel like they were fully recovered, the majority with full depth procedures felt completely healed by 18 months. Being a proactive patient in your own recovery by applying stretching, massage, and acupuncture/acupressure can and will help you recover smoother and more quickly with less complications.

Everyone's experience with this procedure is going to be different. We have different tolerance levels for pain; we use different surgeons who may have slightly different techniques, and some of us have to go back to work sooner rather than later. Everyone's body will heal at a slightly different rate. What might be easy for one person might be difficult for another person. What I hope I have given you in this book are ways that you can speed your recovery and ways that you can approach different problems you might encounter on your own path.

The isolation of this procedure can be difficult for many of us. Hopefully you now know that you are not alone in your pain and recovery. This procedure is deeply fulfilling, and if you ask doctors and surgeons why they work in this specialty field, many of them say that it is because patients are so happy and thankful about the surgery.

I heard a gal who had their surgery 40-plus years ago say once, "When I was first out of surgery, the doctor came to me and handed me a large steel dilator and said to me, 'You have to dilate with this from now on.' Imagine how those early founding women felt having no one to help them through this incredibly profound journey.

As your date nears, even if it is a year away, having a clear set of intentions leading up to your special day will help things go smoothly for you. As a trans woman, I am all-too-aware of intentions; my intention to transition at an older age was stronger than my alcoholism and self-abuse. Our intention gives us strength for our journey. Our intentions give us focus when we may feel lost. In this instance leading up to your date, having positive, clear intentions helps. There can be daily intentions, and/or there may be dreams intentions, life, or goal-oriented intentions. You can turn your intentions into a mantra you repeat daily or when you need some focus. These intentions are a solid platform to help meet goals and lead you to achievements that can elevate you to a desired level of happiness.

This is a simple list of ways that may help you with your personal intentions.

- State your intention or intentions.

- Clarify the intention behind your dreams or goals.

- Write down your intentions, if it helps you.

- Be clear, and make sure the intentions are positive.

- Keep your intentions simple.

- Share your intentions with a close friend or loved one.

- State your intentions out loud to yourself.

- Set your intentions before getting out of bed.

- Shift away from any limiting beliefs.

This is your pledge for your journey, keeping it positive, keep it simple. By clearly stating what you want to experience and achieve through these actions is the nourishment for your goals. Tailor-make your intentions to fit you and all of your unique, flawless beauty. You are about to embark on an adventure that will be scary at times; setting your intentions and knowing that you are not alone on this journey is half the battle.

You got this, girl.

www.ingramcontent.com/pod-product-compliance
Lightning Source LLC
Chambersburg PA
CBHW071019280326
41935CB00011B/1422